Practical occupational
medicine

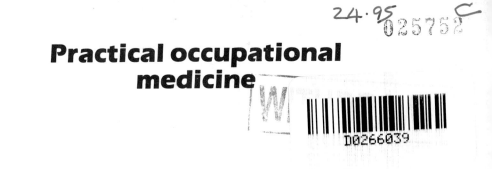

3/94   LIB/LEND/001

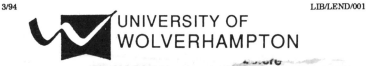

UNIVERSITY OF
WOLVERHAMPTON

Practical occupational medicine

Anthony Seaton MD, FRCP, FRCP(Ed), FFOM,
Professor and Head, Department of Environmental and
Occupational Medicine, University of Aberdeen

Raymond Agius MD, FRCP(Ed), FFOM,
Senior Lecturer in Occupational and Environmental Health,
Department of Public Health Sciences, University of Edinburgh

Elizabeth McCloy BSc, MB, BS, FFOM,
Chief Executive and Director, Civil Service Occupational
Health Service

Denis D'Auria MA, LIM, MD, FFOM,
Chief Medical Adviser, Midland Bank PLC

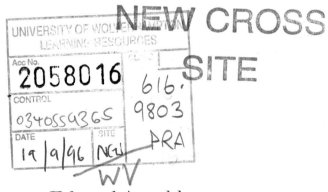
Edward Arnold
A member of the Hodder Headline Group
LONDON   BOSTON   MELBOURNE   AUCKLAND

© 1994 Edward Arnold

First published in Great Britain 1994

Distributed in the Americas by Little, Brown and Company,
34 Beacon Street, Boston, MA 02108

British Library Cataloguing in Publication Data

Seaton, Anthony
  Practical Occupational Medicine
  I. Title
  616.9803

ISBN 0-340-55936-5

Whilst the advice and information in this book is believed to be
true and accurate at the date of going to press, neither the authors
nor the publisher can accept any legal responsibility or liability
for any errors or omissions that may be made. In particular (but
without limiting the generality of the preceding disclaimer) every
effort has been made to check drug dosages; however, it is still
possible that errors have been missed. Furthermore, dosage
schedules are constantly being revised and new side effects
recognised. For these reasons the reader is strongly urged to consult
the drug companies' printed instructions before administering any
of the drugs recommended in this book.

Typeset in 10/12 pt Times by Anneset, Weston-super-Mare, Avon.
Printed in Great Britain for Edward Arnold, a division of Hodder
Headline PLC, 338 Euston Road, London NW1 3BH by St
Edmundsbury Press Ltd, Bury St Edmunds, Suffolk and bound by
Hunter & Foulis Ltd, Edinburgh.

Preface

In recent years there has been an increased awareness by the public of workplace hazards and of the health risks that may be associated with them, and important steps have been taken to simplify and make more effective legislation on health and safety at work. More doctors are becoming involved, fulltime or parttime, in providing advice to industry and to employers on health in relation to the workplace, and there are now several post-graduate professional and vocational courses in the subject. Since, however, occupational medicine has received little emphasis in the curricula of most British medical schools, doctors are often illequipped to take on responsibilities in a specialty with which they have little familiarity.

In our undergraduate and postgraduate teaching we have become aware of the need for an introductory textbook written in such a way as to bridge the gap between normal clinical practice, which is concerned mostly with diagnosis and treatment of disease, and occupational practices which concerns itself with prevention of workrelated disease and with nonpharmacological management of illhealth in relation to the workplace. Common to both types of practice is the ill or atrisk individual, and it is with such people and their management that this book is concerned. We have based the structure of the book on real examples of problems encountered in our practice, problems that may be familiar to our readers but that may nevertheless cause difficulties in management through unfamiliarity with occupational medical practice.

We hope this book will be of value to medical students as a complement to their studies of internal medicine, general practice and public health, and also to general practitioners and other postgraduates taking courses in occupational medicine. Increasingly, nurses are playing an important role in the provision of occupational health services, and we believe it will be of value to them when working for occupational health qualifications. Many established consultants who occasionally see patients suspected of having occupational disease will also find it contains useful, practical information and advice. If in writing it we have conveyed some of our own enthusiasm for a specialty that crosses traditional medical boundaries into other scientific fields and the world of industry, we shall be well satisfied.

Contents

1

The occupational history

Summary

The occupational history should serve two functions – to enable the doctor to detect influences of the patient's work on his or her health, and to allow sensible advice to be given on the effects of the patient's health on future working ability. This chapter describes the important questions to ask in a routine occupational history, about the name of the job, what it involves and what possible relevant hazards it entails. It also describes how to take a more detailed history when work-related disease is suspected or when there is a need to give advice about return to work (or retiral from work) after illness.

Introduction

Every medical student is taught the importance of taking an occupational history, the emphasis of this being on the need to think of occupational causes of disease. However, since in clinical practice such conditions are perceived as being relatively uncommon, the young doctor often forgets this early lesson and simply records the job title of the patient. Indeed, it is quite usual in reviewing hospital or general practice notes to find no reference at all to a patient's occupation. This lack of curiosity about what people spend half of their waking hours doing means that possible subtle influences of work on health are commonly missed by the doctor, and the perception that work-related ill-health is rare is thus reinforced. Furthermore, it results in the doctor being ill-equipped to answer three questions commonly asked by patients, namely, 'should I stay off work?', 'when can I go back to work?' and 'could my work have caused my problem?'.

The occupational history should be taken in such a way as to equip the doctor to judge whether the patient's health has been affected by work and also to decide whether the illness will affect the patient's ability to continue working normally. These two concepts:

- the effects of work on health and
- the effects of health on work

are the basis of occupational medical practice.

Taking the history

This need not be a lengthy procedure. However, it should involve more than recording the job title. Consider, for example, the range of activities covered by the title 'doctor', from a surgeon rushing from blood-spattered operation to out-patients to fevered committee meeting, to a community physician who may spend much of the day planning provision of services and working at a computer. What is necessary is to obtain information on what the patient does at work. The key questions are:

- do you have a job?
- what is it?
- what do you do at work?

and if thought to be relevant:

- do you work with any chemicals, dusts or fumes?
- do you have any problems at work?
- do you have any difficulty doing your work?

The first of these questions may be adapted to the patient's complaint, asking for example about noise, vibration or awkward postures where relevant.

Finally, it is often sensible to ask:

- do you have any other jobs?

Here there is overlap with hobbies and pastimes, which may also be relevant. It is important to know how long the patient has had the job. If it has been for a relatively short period, it is sensible to obtain information about the main work the patient has done previously. In certain circumstances, when a patient presents with a chronic disease or with a cancer, it may be useful to know about jobs done years before.

The job

Case history 1.1

A 30-year old man presented with episodic wheeze and cough. He gave as his occupation 'panel beater', a trade involving the repair of the bodywork of crashed cars. Further questions were therefore directed at the possibility of exposure to sprayed paint and he said that this activity did take place in the garage, but by others and in a specially constructed booth; he was not exposed to the paint. By way of explanation, he was told that some two-part paints contain isocyanates and that these chemicals can cause asthma. He then admitted that he had a second job in which he repaired car bodywork in his own garage at home. He had been using an isocyanate-based paint spray without any exhaust ventilation or respiratory protection! This proved to be the cause of his asthma, and after he had purchased appropriate respiratory protection and ventilation equipment he was able to continue this work without symptoms.

Case history 1.2

A 50-year old lady presented with increasing and severe breathlessness over a period of about 5 years. She looked ill and her chest radiographs showed bilateral upper lobe fibrosis and lower zone emphysema. She had never smoked, and had worked for the same company as a clerical officer for 30 years. She was employed as a clerk but described her current task as operating an industrial camera. This involved a stage during which she dusted exposed plates with a special powder. The work was done in a small room and the powder got everywhere; apparently the service engineer for another machine in the room had complained that the dust kept jamming its works.

Upper lobe fibrosis has relatively few causes, the best known of which is tuberculosis. Accelerated silicosis is a rare cause, and examination of the powder she had been using showed it to be pure crystalline silicon dioxide. This information came too late to help the unfortunate patient, but did allow action to be taken to prevent others suffering the same fate.

These two histories illustrate the importance of obtaining some detail about the work done in someone's job, and also show the difficulties that may lead to an occupational cause being missed. In Chapter 2 we discuss the range of diseases that may have an occupational cause; there is almost no specialty in medicine in which occupational ill-health can be disregarded.

As a doctor becomes more experienced, the process of history taking becomes more economical of time. In busy practice it is usual to record the essentials of the occupational history initially, but to return for further elaboration if the medical history or examination reveals further clues. In taking a medical history always be open-minded about the possibility of environmental causes of disease. Most illness is clearly not wholly genetically determined. Environment therefore must play a part in the aetiology of many diseases; if we do not know the cause of a disease, that does not mean that it cannot be discovered or that a cause does not exist.

In taking a history aimed at investigating the possibility of work-related disease, the relationship between work and exposure is crucial. In acute diseases, such as pneumonitis and allergic alveolitis, a history of recent exposure to a gas or an allergen will be obtained, though this exposure may have been several days previously in the case, say, of exposure to nitrogen dioxide from silage. Variable conditions, such as asthma and some forms of dermatitis, may fluctuate as exposure fluctuates, improving on holidays and at weekends. Conditions such as pneumoconiosis and industrial deafness are usually the consequence of prolonged exposure over several years, although relatively short high intensity exposure may sometimes be responsible. Cancer often is a response to exposure to carcinogens in the distant past, though again usually over a prolonged period. In all these instances, it is helpful to enquire in the history as to whether any of the patient's workmates are known to have suffered similar symptoms or illnesses.

Harmful workplace environments

If occupational disease is suspected, the occupational history should include an attempt to assess the patient's exposure to risk. This is done in two steps:

- what has the patient been exposed to?
  and
- to how much?

Of course, the provisional diagnosis of occupational disease will not have been made unless the occupational and medical histories provided appropriate clues. These clues are then followed up by questions about likely causes of the syndrome and about the patient's working practices in relation to the suspect cause.

Case history 1.3

A 55-year old man presented with progressive difficulty with arm and leg coordination over some four years. This had eventually forced him to retire from his job, since when the symptoms had ceased to progress, although they remained very disabling. He gave his job as an armaments fitter. Examination showed classical signs of cerebellar ataxia, without evidence of disease of other parts of the nervous system. Investigations led to the diagnosis of cerebellar degeneration, confirmed by computerized tomography.

The patient himself, puzzling about the cause of his disease, joined a self-help group and learned that the condition could sometimes be caused by the drug phenytoin. He told his doctor that this led him to consider the possibility that chemicals at his work had been responsible. A detailed occupational history revealed that for 10 years he had worked in a relatively confined space, without exhaust ventilation, disassembling missiles. After stripping these down, he spent about three hours each day cleaning their parts with solvents, using a rag onto which he poured the solvent from an open tin. Much of this cleaning work took place at face level. He wore no protective gloves or respirator. Subsequent measurements of exposure levels showed them to be considerably in excess of the appropriate hygiene standards during this work. Although workplace exposure to the solvents in question had not previously been shown to cause neurological damage, by analogy with neurological syndromes in glue-sniffers, it seemed very likely that his disease was in fact due to his very high and prolonged workplace exposures. This opinion received some support from a small but definite subsequent clinical improvement after exposure had ceased for about a year.

The above case history illustrates an important point. From time to time patients may present with disease that has not previously been described in relation to the substances they are exposed to at work. An open mind should be kept, since occasionally, as in this case, the occupational history reveals exposures very much in excess of what would normally have been expected – this patient used solvents for at least 15 hours each week and absorbed them both through his lungs and his skin. It should also be borne in mind that individuals differ in susceptibility to harmful substances; this is particularly true in the case of asthma and dermatitis, and will be discussed further in Chapters 2 and 3.

The sensible way to take a semi-quantitative occupational exposure history is to obtain the patient's account of a typical day – What time do you go to work? What do you do when you get in? How long do you do it for? Do any dusts or fumes come off? Do you handle any chemicals? . . . and so on, until the end of the shift. Remember to ask about protective clothing and equipment and for how long the job has been done. This sort of history, which is of course only necessary when an occupational disease is suspected, allows an estimate to be made of cumulative exposure which can subsequently be enhanced by actual workplace measurements (see Chapter 3).

A careful structured occupational history may sometimes reveal a totally unexpected cause.

Case history 1.4

A patient was cleaning a heat exchanger in a potato crisp factory when he developed a severe attack of asthma, the first he had ever had. He had to go home, where he recovered after treatment by his doctor, but he got a similar attack, also when in the vicinity of the heat exchanger, the next day. Several subsequent attacks occurred at work and he arrived at the view that he had occupational asthma, attributing it to something in the heat exchanger and to chemicals used as fungicides on the potatoes he had to handle.

The original occupational history revealed that he had very little contact with the potatoes and that his work in the heat exchanger had involved exposure to dust which was almost certainly carbon. There seemed to be no plausible antigen. However, using the technique described above, it transpired that his first task on entering the factory was to sweep out the joiners' workshop. Thereafter he went on to other labouring jobs of a more or less innocuous nature, of which cleaning the heat exchanger had been one. The joiners had been using red cedar, a wood to the dust of which he had been exposed in a previous job as a joiner himself. He proved to have red cedar allergy, and this allowed steps to be taken to prevent further trouble.

Protective measures taken

When occupational disease is suspected, the history is not complete without an assessment of the adequacy of any preventive measures. This is particularly so in medico-legal practice, where a patient may find the employer claiming that the worker's injury or illness was contributed to by a failure to protect him or herself. The principles of protection are discussed in Chapter 5, but essentially they are based on an understanding that risks to health should, as far as is reasonably practicable, be designed out. Thus, relatively safe substances should have preference over harmful ones, harmful substances should not come into contact with individuals and finally, personal protection should be provided when necessary. The occupational history should reveal whether these criteria were observed and also when. Remember that harmful substances may enter the body by the lungs, skin or alimentary tract.

Sometimes a well-known occupational disease may occur in spite of adequate precautions being taken, because particular groups of workers or individuals escape the protective net.

Case history 1.5

Bladder cancer is a well-known hazard of workers exposed to certain organic dyes, and for this reason the manufacturers are particularly careful to protect their workers by enclosure of processes and provision of protective clothing and changing facilities. One patient with the disease, however, had spent many years working for an engineering company as a fitter. His company had a contract to service and repair the machinery at the dye factory. He therefore had to penetrate the protective barriers and became regularly soaked in the chemicals when doing his work. By an oversight, the company had not provided him, as an outside worker, with the protective clothing and facilities enjoyed by the company's employees, and consequently he was exposed by skin contact to hazardous amounts of bladder carcinogens.

Several lessons arise from this case history. First, the term 'fitter' covers a multitude of jobs and workplaces, but usually means the worker will be employed when something needs repairing. This is often a dangerous time, as the protective barriers are down and harmful substances may be present. Second, an employer is responsible for the health and safety of all on the worksite, not just the direct employees, but also contractors and visitors. Third, old-fashioned occupational diseases still occur. The reason they are old-fashioned is that precautions have generally been taken to prevent them – if people forget about these precautions, the diseases come back.

In enquiring about protective measures in the occupational history, ask about:

- enclosure of the process and segregation from it
- ventilation
- protective clothing, respirators, hearing protection, etc.
- what happens when the process is serviced or repaired
- information provided on hazards
- education given to workers on protecting themselves.

Assessing fitness for the job

The more frequent need for an occupational history is to assess the fitness of a patient for return to work. It is never sufficient to assume the level of activity in a job; a lorry driver, for example, is usually responsible for loading and unloading his vehicle, whereas a miner may sometimes ride to the coalface and spend his day sitting on a cutting or drilling machine. Most workers learn the most physically economical method of doing their job, while some severely impaired individuals manage a demanding job by relying on the support of fitter colleagues. A great deal of time is lost from industry, and thus much money spent unproductively, as a result of sickness absence (see Chapter 7). A doctor has a responsibility both to the patient and to the employer in this respect, and should not keep patients off work needlessly. Knowledge of the demands of the job will often help in planning appropriate rehabilitative measures.

Case history 1.6

> An auxiliary nurse had a car crash, causing a whiplash type of neck injury. She had no neurological problems, but developed stiffness and pains in her neck and shoulders. She worked on a geriatric assessment ward, and most of her day was spent assisting patients out of bed and encouraging their mobility. All of this work involved moderately vigorous arm activity. Rehabilitation was planned to encourage recovery of upper limb mobility by swimming exercise, and within two weeks of starting the programme she was able to return to supervised duties on the ward.

In order to make a realistic assessment of the demands of a job when considering return to work, a similar occupational history to that for assessing exposure is required. However, there are some differences. Most notably, for many people the problems of getting back to work after illness are as much related to travel to and from work as to the demands of the job. Remember to ask what time the patient has to get up in the morning and how he or she gets to and from work. An hour or two each day in the rush hour of London's Underground is considerably more stressful, both physically and psychologically, than many jobs. In addition, for many low-paid workers a tiring shift pattern and regular overtime are an inescapable part of the job, making return to full-time work more difficult. Finally, ask whether the patient enjoys the job. The attentions of macho managers and bullying colleagues can make the lives of some workers miserable, while, equally, financial pressures and production targets can be strong factors in decisions about when managers should return to work.

The patient is usually the best judge of when he or she is ready to return to work. However, the doctor who has some knowledge of the implications of the diagnosis and its prognosis must provide guidance, based on the patient's account of the job. Some large companies have rehabilitation programmes, while small companies can often provide appropriate gradual reintroduction to work if asked. These matters are discussed further in Chapter 8.

2

Work-related diseases

Summary

Whatever your specialty, you may come across disease related to occupation. The most common of these are stress reactions presenting to the general practitioner, psychiatrist or physician, and dermatitis presenting to the general practitioner and the dermatologist. Almost as frequent are orthopaedic complaints – overuse syndromes in the arm and back problems. The general surgeon may see Raynaud's syndrome caused by vibrating tools, the ear, nose and throat (ENT) surgeon tinnitus and deafness due to noise, and the gynaecologist and endocrinologist reproductive problems caused by chemicals. The chest physician can expect to see occupational lung diseases regularly and the renal physician kidney and bladder problems caused by chemicals occasionally. The general practitioner will see any of these, together with an array of non-specific symptoms that may be related to the workplace.

This chapter describes the broad range of occupational diseases, as far as possible according to the features they present to the general practitioner or hospital doctor. Their diagnosis usually depends on the doctor being alert to the possibility of an occupational cause and being able to take an appropriate occupational history.

Introduction

The classical occupational diseases were described during the Industrial Revolution. Several of the earliest to be recognized were cancers – scrotal cancer in chimney sweeps, lung cancer in metal miners, bladder cancer in aniline dye workers and skin cancer in oil shale refiners. Other almost equally serious conditions were also common in the industrial world at the turn of the century – silicosis, lead and arsenic poisoning, and the effects of radiation, for example. This pattern has now changed, metal poisonings and the classical occupational cancers having largely been eliminated in the developed world, pneumoconioses being under partial control, and diseases due to pesticides, asbestos and other chemicals having taken their place. In addition, the type of work people do has led to recognition of a different spectrum of less dramatic but often very troublesome and chronic conditions – dermatitis, vibration injury and deafness, locomotor problems, especially related to the spine, and overuse injury such as tenosynovitis. Finally, psychological disease of the anxiety-depression type is commonly related, at least in part, to problems in the workplace.

Whether occupational disease is becoming more or less common is impossible to say in the absence of good statistics. Mortality from some serious diseases, such as bladder cancer in dye and rubber workers, has clearly declined as has metal poisoning. Worldwide, pesticide poisoning is an important cause of death and less severe episodes are not uncommon in the West. Death rates from mesothelioma due to asbestos exposure from the 1940s to 1970s continue to rise, while newly described diseases, such as hepatic angiosarcoma in vinyl chloride workers, appear in a cluster and then decline as preventive action is taken. In Britain, statistics are published by the Health and Safety Executive on notifications of occupational disease from various sources, by the Registrars General on causes of death, and as a result of informal reporting procedures such as those for occupational respiratory and haematological disorders. In addition, statistics on successful claims for Industrial Injuries Benefit give some indication of the incidence of certain recognized (or 'prescribed') diseases. This latter source, although limited to people who have felt it necessary to make a claim and have then been assessed as disabled, is currently the most useful source for studying trends over time. These sources are summarized in Table 2.1, and some further information is given in Appendix 1.

The size of the problem

Since the data are patchy and incomplete, only a very rough estimate of the size of the problem may be arrived at, and that only for certain conditions.

In terms of disability, approximately 185,000 people are currently in receipt of benefits for industrial injury in the UK. Of these, about 150,000 suffered an industrial accident and the rest have occupational deafness or other occupational diseases. These figures are undoubtedly biased by fashions in making claims, thus providing a truer picture at present of the prevalence of deafness than, say, of vibration injury or upper limb strain disorders. Pneumoconioses due to coal (approximately 300 cases per annum) and silica (approximately 80 cases per annum) have been declining slowly, though it should be noted that there has been a comparable decline in the numbers of people at risk in the relevant industries. Asbestos diseases have continued to rise. Mesothelioma deaths, of which about 90 per cent are attributable to occupational exposure, had reached 860 in 1988, in which year 202 people received disablement benefit for asbestosis. About 60 people with asbestosis die each year of lung cancer, though the actual incidence of asbestos-related lung cancer is probably higher than this. Other recognized occupational cancers account for some 30 deaths

Table 2.1 Sources of information on occupational disease in the UK

Source	Type of Information
Registrars General	Causes of death – limited to fatal and serious conditions. Biased by diagnostic habits of doctors
Department of Social Security	Disablement awards – limited to prescribed diseases and to people who have applied and are disabled
Department of Employment (Health and Safety Executive)	Reported diseases – limited to listed diseases and biased by reporting habits of employers
Sampling of GP referrals or accident and emergency attendances by Health and Safety Executive	Occasional studies to estimate annual incidence of specific diseases, confined so far to dermatitis and workplace poisonings
Worker surveillance under specific regulations (Health and Safety Executive)	Confined to workers exposed to lead, ionising radiation and asbestos. Detailed information available on registered workers
Surveillance schemes by NHS consultants and occupational physicians	Confined to respiratory and haematological diseases seen by participants since 1989. Gives the most complete information available; data on trends will soon be available

per annum, though estimates of the likely number of cases in which occupation has contributed to cancer death suggest that (including asbestos cancer and mesothelioma) perhaps 5000 occur each year.

Of the less dramatic conditions, some 500 new cases of occupational asthma are now being reported each year. Surveys suggest that there may be about 60,000 patients with occupational dermatitis presenting to general practitioners annually, although only about 300 of these seem to be sufficiently severe to receive disablement benefit each year. About 1500 people each year receive benefits for industrial deafness and some 800 for upper limb strain disorders. Again, those receiving benefit are clearly the tip of a large iceberg, and a recent survey of 60,000 households (the 1990 Labour Force Survey) has shown that work-related locomotor and psychological illness were afflicting over 600,000 people in one year. Some figures are shown in Appendix 1.

Causes and targets

Hazards and risks

Consider a workplace environment with which all doctors and clinical students are familiar, the hospital. Most people working within it will not have thought of it as a particularly hazardous environment, at least to themselves (Fig. 2.1). The word hazard, derived from the Arabic for a gaming die, implies the potential to cause harm. The likelihood of harm occurring is called the risk, a concept that can be quantified (Fig. 2.2). These complementary meanings of words which are often used synonymously are important in occupational medicine, since a hazardous substance may need to be used, but can often be used in a way that substantially reduces the risk to the individuals concerned. How might hazards in the hospital environment be classified? What risks, and to whom, do they imply?

Table 2.2 gives a general classification of hazards such as can be applied to any workplace. Let us consider these in relation to the job of, say, house surgeon. First, psychological. Here, the demands of the job may be considerable, especially in the first month or two. Long hours, an endless series of tasks, the anxiety of personal responsibility for the health of others, often the inability to complete one task before another is imposed . . . .

Such heavy psychological stresses may be compounded by difficult relationships with senior colleagues and nursing staff, who may appear not to appreciate the problems of the young doctor. The environment may also be unsatisfactory – poor recreational facilities, a bedroom close to a busy main road, poor catering, and so on. It is clear that such hazards entail a high risk of psychological problems; the thing that keeps most house surgeons going is the knowledge that it will only be as bad as that for a year. This, however, is not the case with other stressful and less well-paid jobs, such as the hospital

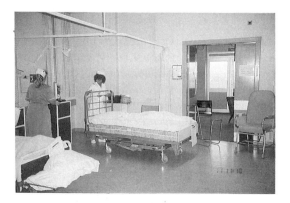

Fig. 2.1   A familiar environment

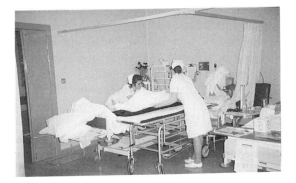

Fig. 2.2   The risk of back injury in nurses can be measured

Table 2.2   A classification of hazards

Physical	Noise and vibration
	Heat and cold
	Radiation
	Trauma and loads
Chemical, including minerals	Gases, vapours and aerosols
	Liquids
	Solids
Biological	Infectious agents
	Allergenic particles
Psychological	Interpersonal relationships
	Environmental stressors
	Demands of the job

switchboard operators. Nor is it a reason for taking no action to ameliorate the situation.

Next, physical hazards. Here the house surgeon is at smaller risk. While many hospitals are noisy and overheated, these factors do not normally approach levels sufficient to cause deafness or heat stroke (though there are exceptions – the boiler room and laundry can be very noisy and heat stress may occur in certain operating theatres). There is, of course, a small risk if lasers are used or if the doctor is exposed to ionizing radiation, but such well-recognized hazards are normally controlled very carefully. The most important physical risk to the house surgeon is trauma – assault by a patient or relative is not uncommon, and accidental injury by a knife or needle still occurs regrettably frequently. Awkward postures, in putting up drips or assisting at operations, may also contribute to accident or injury.

Chemical hazards might be thought to be unimportant. Nevertheless some such as anaesthetic gases and cytotoxic drugs are present, though they usually constitute a greater threat to nurses. Sensitization to glutaraldehyde used in sterilizing endoscopes or to chemicals in rubber gloves may occur, as may skin allergies to handling some drugs or to substances used for scrubbing up. Mineral hazards are clearly almost negligible as risks to hospital doctors, though nickel in surgical instruments has in the past caused dermatitis. Asbestos in lagging in hospital ducts is only a threat to the engineering staff.

Biological hazards are well recognized in hospitals. The classical examples, tuberculosis and streptococcal septicaemia, have now largely been prevented. Though the risks are much smaller than was the pre-chemotherapy risk of tuberculosis, Hepatitis B and HIV infection have now taken over as potential infective causes of death in doctors. Preventive measures in hospitals should ensure that these risks are kept to a minimum. The other important infective hazard in modern hospitals is Legionnaire's disease, though this seems more inclined to afflict patients and visitors, perhaps because of pre-existing susceptibility, than young doctors. Again, the risk is able to be reduced substantially by appropriate preventive action.

This example serves to illustrate the operation of hazard and risk in a familiar environment. In terms of risk, the house surgeon may be expected to suffer periods of anxiety and depression, at least until effective action is taken to ameliorate working conditions. The more susceptible will suffer serious psychological illness. Many house surgeons (and nurses) will be assaulted by a patient or by a drunk in the Casualty Department. Risks of cuts and needlestick injury are high (Fig. 2.3), though fortunately most are minor; nevertheless, the HIV epidemic means that in the future none will be able to be regarded as trivial even though the risk of infection from a single such injury remains very low. Chemical and other risks may be regarded as very low in most circumstances. All these risks are able to be reduced by appropriate preventive action. Rather than accepting them as necessary accompaniments of the job, the occupational physician should take

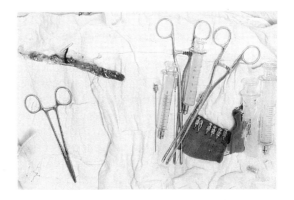

Fig. 2.3   A day's collection of 'sharps' from the hospital laundry

active steps to promote awareness of risk and to develop strategy to reduce it. This is considered further in Chapter 5.

The targets of injury

The remainder of this chapter describes the main syndromes of occupational disease, considered as far as practicable from the point of view of the presenting features. These features are usually common to many different conditions, non-occupational as well as occupational, and the aim of the chapter is to alert the reader to the possibility of occupational causes. The diseases have been grouped generally according to organ systems, and reflect those systems which are most usually the target of occupational disease. Thus, the skin and the lung, both in direct contact with the outside environment, feature prominently, as does the locomotor system as the site of much traumatic injury. The ear and eye may also be affected quite commonly at work by physical hazards. Less commonly, absorbed chemical substances may injure the brain and nervous system, or the liver and urinary tract in the process of biotransformation and excretion.

Substances and physical hazards in the workplace may injure the body by any of the range of known mechanisms – inflammatory reactions due to trauma, infection, allergy and other cellular responses to foreign particles, interference with normal metabolism by chemicals, initiation or promotion of neoplastic change by carcinogens, other consequences of genotoxicity, and the subtle changes in neuro-endocrine function associated with adverse psychological environments leading to stress reactions.

Skin disease

The main symptoms of occupational, as of other sorts of skin disease are soreness, itch, the appearance of a rash or lump, and occasionally pigmentary changes. Occupational causes can evoke a wide range of pathological responses, but the site of the lesion is of great importance in making the diagnosis, since in all cases it occurs at least initially at the site of contact with the offending agent. Equally important is a careful history of the evolution of the lesion and of chemicals and materials with which the patient comes into contact. Finally, it is essential to ask if others in the workplace have similar problems – occupational skin disease often occurs in clusters.

Contact dermatitis

This is the most common occupational disease seen in practice, and may be of irritant or allergic types (Fig. 2.4).

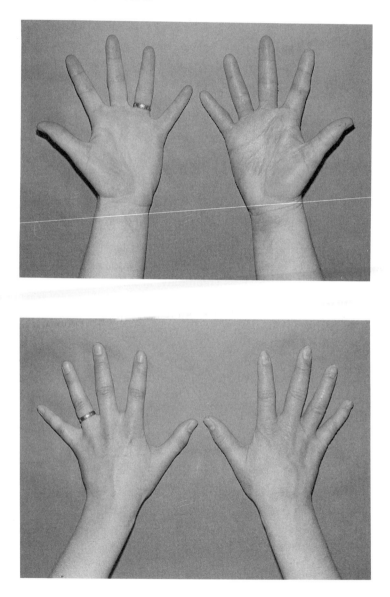

Fig. 2.4   Dermatitis of the right hand in a nurse. The unilateral distribution resulted from her using a rubber surgical glove on her right hand for certain cleaning duties

Case history 2.1

Sore itchy hands were reported in two technicians working in a medical school. In one, the backs and sides of the fingers were red and sore with some fissuring. In the other the fingers were red, swollen and itchy and the technician said that when it was bad her eyelids swelled up and itched also. Both had to wear rubber gloves frequently for their work with cell cultures and tissue slices. In the first case, the cause was frequent washing and scrubbing of the skin of the hands, an irritant dermatitis, while in the second sensitization to the rubber gloves (or rather to one of the chemicals added to the latex in their manufacture) had occurred – an allergic dermatitis. The first was treated by modifying the washing procedure and the second by changing to non-allergenic vinyl gloves.

Both types of contact dermatitis may become chronic if the cause is not identified and eliminated. Allergic dermatitis is an example of a Type 4 immunological reaction involving sensitized T-lymphocytes. It commonly spreads to other parts of the skin and may even present as a widespread eczematous rash. It usually occurs after several weeks' exposure to the sensitizing agent, though faster responses to potent sensitizers do occur. Some of the important causes and occupations in which contact dermatitis occurs are shown in Table 2.3.

Skin infections and infestations

Itchy eruptions may be due to the scabies mite or to flea bites. The first is a risk of health care workers, the second of people in contact particularly with cats. Mites from stored vegetable matter, especially grain, and from bird droppings may occasionally cause itchy lesions. All these reactions are due to a sensitivity reaction to substances excreted or injected by the arthropod.

Table 2.3   Common causes of contact dermatitis

Cause	Occupations at risk
Irritant	
Cement*	Building
Oils	Operating machinery
Solvents	Painting, cleaning
Detergents	Housework, hairdressing, cleaning
Fibre glass	Insulation, building
Allergic	
Rubber gloves	Surgeons, technicians, nurses
Epoxy resin hardeners	Electrical manufacture, joinery,
	Repair work, painters
Colophony	Soldering, lacquering, adhesives
Cobalt	Glass, pottery manufacture,
	Hard metal industry
Nickel	Electroplaters, use of metal tools
Formaldehyde,	
glutaraldehyde	Nurses, laboratory technicians
Dyes, perms	Hairdressing
Plants (e.g. primula)	Horticulture, florists
Wood (especially hardwoods)	Joiners, carpenters

Note   * May also cause allergic dermatitis if it contains chrome

Skin infections are less common, apart from fungal infections of the feet transmitted in communal shower facilities such as at coalmines. A few exotic infections may be seen.

Case history 2.2

A young surgical registrar presented at the Occupational Health Department with a non-tender lump on her finger *(Fig. 2.5)*. She informed the doctor that she had orf, a pox virus lesion, acquired the previous weekend during which she had helped her parents with the lambing. In particular she had hand-fed one lamb that had severe buccal ulceration. Care was taken to prevent her uncovered hand coming into contact with patients and she was prohibited from operating until the lesion had evolved through ulcerative and granulomatous stages to healing over the subsequent month.

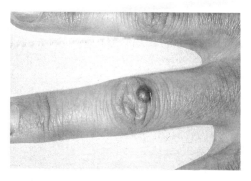

Fig. 2.5   Early lesion of orf in a hospital registrar

Anthrax, which also presents with a boil-like lesion, though in this case associated with systemic illness, is now quite rare. Less rare is erysipeloid, an infection caused by *Erysipelothrix rhusiopathiae* a Gram-positive bacillus. It causes a spreading red, itchy patch round a skin scratch or laceration, and may produce systemic malaise, lymphadenopathy and even septicaemia and endocarditis. It afflicts people handling animals or their carcases, most commonly fish, which gives it its common name of fish handlers' disease.

Pigmentary changes

Exposure to tar and similar substances, as in road work or roofing, and to certain plants such as fennel and dill, can cause photosensitization and unexpected sunburn. So can inadvertent exposure to ultra-violet light.

Case history 2.3

A group of workers in a sausage factory came to the attention of the Health and Safety Executive's doctor because of complaints of sunburn on arms and faces at work. No chemical exposure was taking place but, in common with many food-processing factories, there were insect traps which used ultra-violet (UV) light as an attractant. Examination of these lights showed that they had been fitted, by mistake, with bulbs emitting UV-C rather than UV-A. UV-C is used as a method of killing airborne bacteria, and has high photon energy. It is absorbed by the superficial layers of the skin where it causes burning.

Hyperpigmentation of the skin may be a consequence of prolonged exposure to tar products, dyes, heavy metals and chlorinated hydrocarbons. Loss of pigmentation, vitiligo, of a patchy sort is caused by exposure to certain chemicals used in adhesives and disinfectants, most notably hydroquinone and para substituted phenols (Fig. 2.6).

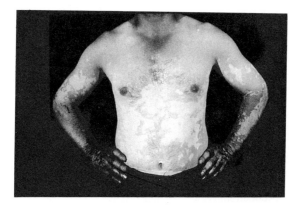

Fig. 2.6 Vitiligo caused by exposure to phenolic compounds. (Courtesy of Dr C.J. Stevenson)

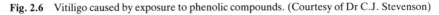

Spots

Acne may occasionally be a consequence of workplace exposure. Oils and oil mists may cause such lesions, especially on the arms. A severe form, chloracne, with itchy cystic lesions that often progress to scarring and affect particularly the face, is caused by exposure to chlorinated biphenyls used in the electrical industry. Other chlorinated aromatic compounds may cause the same condition.

Scleroderma

Occasionally sclerodermatous changes may be seen in patients as a result of occupational exposure. When confined to the hands and associated with Raynaud's syndrome and erosion of the terminal phalanges, a syndrome known as acro-osteolysis, it is caused by high levels of exposure to vinyl chloride in PVC production. Scleroderma, sometimes associated with systemic sclerosis, is also a risk of prolonged exposure to quartz and may accompany silicosis.

Lung disease

The usual presentation of patients with occupational lung disease is no different from that of patients with non-occupational disease with one or other of breathlessness, persistent cough, chest pain, or the report of an abnormal chest radiograph. Occasionally they may present with anxiety that they are being harmed by something at work. Most of the well-known syndromes of lung disease have one or more occupational causes (Table 2.4). The key to the detection of these is the occupational history, as outlined in Chapter 1.

Occupational asthma

Occupational asthma is reported in about 500 people each year in Britain, and is estimated to occur up to three times as commonly as this. The diagnosis is easily missed, unless the key questions are asked of all new asthmatic patients:

- Does the wheeze change at weekends or on holiday?
- Does anything at work affect your chest?

Table 2.4   Some occupational causes of lung disease

Syndrome	Main Causes
Asthma	Animals, hard woods, grains
	epoxy resins, isocyanates etc.
Allergic alveolitis	Mouldy hay, fungi and actinomycetes
Chronic bronchitis/ emphysema	Cigarette smoke, coal dust, cadmium
Bronchial carcinoma	Radiation, chloromethyl ethers, asbestos
Nodular or diffuse fibrosis	Silica, coal, asbestos
Sarcoidosis	Beryllium
Tuberculosis	*M. tuberculosis*
	(Health care workers)
Pneumonitis	Toxic gases, cadmium fumes
Pneumonia	*Legionella sp*
Pleural fibrosis	Asbestos, silica
Mesothelioma	Asbestos

Case history 2.4

A 50 year-old man complained of episodic but increasing wheeze and shortness of breath over about a year. The symptoms were typically asthmatic and he was instructed in appropriate treatment, after he had denied knowledge of any provocative factors. His work sounded innocuous, as a labourer in a washing machine factory. However, no sooner was he out of the clinic than his wife came in, insisting that his work was to blame. This uninvited intervention led to the discovery that isocyanates were being used in the factory, and this proved to be the cause of his disease. His symptoms remitted when he was redeployed.

Occupational asthma starts after the patient has started the job, the interval being variable. At first intermittent and mild, with continuous exposure it tends to become more persistent and severe. Often there is a history of worsening through the week, partial relief at weekends and more complete relief on holidays. After several months of symptoms, the asthma may become intractable. While it is still relatively mild, the usual diurnal pattern is of onset an hour or two into the shift, progressively worsening during the day and, often, attacks in the night. If exposure to the sensitizing agent is intermittent, the asthma usually reflects this, though one exposure may sometimes lead to recurrent attacks over several days.

Once the condition has been diagnosed and exposure prevented the asthma usually remits. If, however, it has become chronic this remission may take months and may never be complete. Persistent chronic asthma is an occasional consequence. Once sensitized, patients' future exposure should be controlled very carefully, as severe recurrence may occur. Deaths have been reported in relation to re-exposure to some chemical substances.

The main causes of occupational asthma are given in Table 2.5. They divide into classical protein antigens and low molecular weight chemicals. The former elicit an IgE-mediated allergic reaction, as do some of the chemicals by the formation of haptens. Other chemicals cause indistinguishable disease, but without the intervention of IgE, and the mechanisms of sensitization remain unknown. The pathophysiology of occupational asthma, with mediator-induced bronchial mucosal eosinophilic inflammation and oedema, and airway smooth muscle constriction, does not differ from that of classical asthma.

Certain people may be predisposed to occupational asthma. Atopy, an inherited tendency to produce excessive levels of IgE in response to exposure to organic antigen (the gene being sited on the short arm of chromosome 11), makes an individual more liable to develop symptoms if exposed to protein antigens. Cigarette smoking also increases the likelihood of sensitization to antigen, perhaps through increasing the permeability of airway mucosa to inhaled antigen and thus allowing it greater access to submucosal T lymphocytes. The extent to which these two factors should be taken into

Table 2.5   Some important causes of occupational asthma

Cause	Typical jobs
Animal	
Cats, dogs, horses	Veterinary work
Grain mites	Farming
Insects	Research
Molluscs	Seafood preparation
Rodents	Laboratory, research
Vegetable	
Beans	Food production
Flour, grains	Milling, baking
Gums	Food production
Henna	Hairdressing
Pine resin (colophony)	Soldering, adhesives
Wood (esp. hardwoods)	Joinery, carpentry
Microbial	
B subtilis enzymes	Detergent manufacture
Fungal antigens	Biotechnology, Laboratory, farming
Pharmaceutical	
Cephalosporins	Pharmaceutical industry
Ipecacuanha	
Ispaghula	
Methyldopa	
Penicillins	
Piperazine	
Spiramycin	
TetracyclineB	
Chemical	
Acid anhydrides	Epoxy resin use (adhesives, paints)
Aluminium fumes	Smelting
Amines	Epoxy resin use
Azodicarbonamide	Plastics manufacture
Chromates	Plating, metallurgy
Cobalt	Hard metal work, metallurgy
Diisocyanates	Polyurethane paints, varnishes
Formaldehyde, glutaraldehyde	Disinfectants in hospitals
Nickel salts	Plating, metallurgy
Organic dyes	Dyeing (e.g. woollens)
Perchlorates/phosphates	Hairdressing
Platinum salts	Refining, metallurgy

account in preventing occupational asthma will vary from individual to individual and from industry to industry. Where the sensitizer is potent, it may be sensible to screen out smokers and people with clinical manifestations of atopy. However, it is rarely necessary or desirable to exclude people from work simply on the basis of positive skin tests (see Chapter 5).

Bronchial carcinoma

Lung cancer has become such a common disease, killing some 37,000 people each year in the UK, and is so clearly associated with smoking that we rarely think of other causes. It is worth remembering that the first cause, described in 1879, was with work in metal mines, subsequently shown to be due to ionizing radiation.

Case history 2.5

In 1961 a man of 34 presented to his doctor with haemoptysis. He had never smoked. Nevertheless, he proved to have an oat cell carcinoma of the bronchus. Over the next 20 years, 11 other men aged between 41 and 67 also died of rapidly progressive undifferentiated carcinomas of the bronchus. Only 7 had been smokers but all had worked for the same chemical company making ion-exchange resins, a notoriously dirty and smelly outfit. No doctors made the connection, but the trade union at the factory found out that one of the chemicals used was bischloromethyl ether. This had been found to be one of the most potent causes of bronchial carcinoma, in rats in 1967 and shortly thereafter in humans. To date, some 16 men from this small factory have died of anaplastic lung cancer.

This sad story illustrates an important general point. If a patient presents with a rare cancer, or a common cancer in unusual circumstances (in this case, oat cell carcinoma in a young non-smoker) always suspect an environmental or occupational cause. Moreover, if someone with cancer has worked in the 'chemical' industry, make further enquiries. Known occupational causes of lung cancer are listed in Table 2.6. In addition to these, there is some evidence

Table 2.6 Known occupational causes of bronchial carcinoma

Cause	Some occupations
Arsenic trioxide, arsenites	Smelting, pesticide use
Asbestos	Insulation, asbestos textiles
Dichromates	Manufacture from chrome ore
Bischloromethyl ether	Ion exchange resin manufacture
Mustard gas	Weapons manufacture
Nickel subsulphide	Refining of nickel from ore
Radiation (radon gas)	Uranium and other metal mining

that patients with silicosis have an elevated risk.

There are no features which distinguish occupational lung cancer from the disease associated with cigarette smoking. If an asbestos worker develops lung cancer, it is normally assumed to be related to his asbestos exposure if he also has asbestosis. If not, the likelihood of it being due to asbestos depends on the severity (duration × level) of exposure; asbestos exposure and smoking interact to increase risk of the disease. Radiation and other causes probably add to the risks from smoking. Whereas smokers generally develop lung cancer relatively late in life, those who have been exposed to chemical carcinogens often develop the disease rather earlier. In the case of chloromethyl ethers, the peak incidence has been about 10 years after the start of the exposure.

Acute attacks of breathlessness

An acute attack of breathlessness is most commonly due to asthma or left ventricular failure. Occasionally, however, a patient presents a similar clinical picture without signs of cardiac disease or severe airflow obstruction. The presence of repetitive crackles in inspiration and a tachycardia will often mislead the doctor into thinking, in spite of a normal cardiograph, that left ventricular disease is the cause, and sometimes the chest radiograph may support this diagnosis by showing the appearances of pulmonary oedema (but without Kerley B lines). Two occupational diseases may cause this syndrome – acute allergic alveolitis and inhalation of toxic gas.

Case history 2.6

A 30 year-old farmer was admitted to hospital during the autumn with severe breathlessness of 4 hours' duration. He was cyanosed, tachypnoeic and had a pulse rate of 120. Repetitive inspiratory crackles were audible through both lungs. The cardiograph was normal, chest film showed bilateral pulmonary oedema and peak flow rate was normal at 500 l/min. Blood gases showed hypoxaemia and a low pCO_2. His doctor had given him intravenous diuretics without improvement. From his history it was found that he had spent the previous day ploughing a very dusty field and making silage. The silage had been stacked in a shallow pit in an open-sided barn rather than in a tower (Fig. 2.7). A clinical diagnosis of silo-fillers' lung (acute nitrogen dioxide poisoning) was made and he was treated with steroids, with slow improvement over 2 weeks. Over the course of this period, serology for Mycoplasma pneumoniae and farmers' lung organisms was negative, but a needle lung biopsy showed a granulomatous centriacinar inflammation diagnostic of acute allergic alveolitis. Investigation of his farm showed no nitrogen dioxide being given off by the silage, but large numbers of spores of Micropolyspora faeni in the soil of the ploughed field. Serology to this organism subsequently became positive.

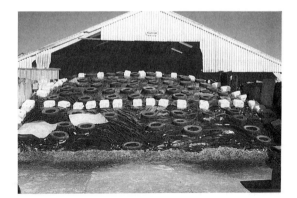

Fig. 2.7   An open-air silage heap. Any gas given off will be rapidly dispersed

This very unusual case illustrates the diagnostic difficulty that may arise with acute non-cardiac breathlessness. Acute allergic alveolitis and pulmonary oedema due to gas inhalation often present in the same way, several hours after exposure to spores or gas, causing similar symptoms and clinical and radiological signs. They also mimic severe viral, mycoplasmal or similar pneumonias. Once again, the history of work done several hours before onset should give the clue. Acute exposure to irritant gas, such as chlorine or sulphur dioxide, is of course always noticed by the patient. However, less irritant gas, such as NO_2 or high concentrations of hydrogen sulphide (which is a chemical asphyxiant), may not be appreciated as possible causes of subsequent breathlessness. Farmers are usually aware of the dangers from mouldy hay, but other workers exposed to high concentrations of fungal spores may not appreciate the risk. Acute allergic alveolitis has been described most frequently in farmers feeding cattle with hay, workers turning barley in whisky production, mushroom workers, and people exposed to fungal-containing dusts in sawmills. In addition, several episodes of allergic alveolitis have been described following exposure to isocyanates. Although many other causes of allergic alveolitis have been described, individual episodes seem to be relatively uncommon, only about 100 being reported in Britain each year. On the other hand, acute episodes of toxic gas inhalation occur relatively frequently, though fortunately few cause serious illness. Approximately 300 are reported in Britain annually.

It should be noted that allergic alveolitis may present in a more insidious form and may progress to chronic pulmonary fibrosis – see next section. Pulmonary oedema secondary to toxic gas inhalation usually resolves spontaneously, though there is evidence that some patients may subsequently develop chronic airflow obstruction.

Chronic breathlessness

Chronic, steadily worsening breathlessness is usually caused by irreversible or partly reversible airflow obstruction, cigarette smoking being the main cause. Less commonly, restrictive lung disease usually due to pulmonary fibrosis is responsible. Occupational factors may be involved in either of these syndromes.

Non-asthmatic chronic airflow obstruction is usually caused pathologically by emphysema, though occasionally narrowing of small airways may be responsible. There is some evidence that exposure to high levels of dust in workplaces, especially coalmines, may contribute to the development of emphysema and airflow obstruction, and it is plausible that many dusts and gases, inhaled in excessive amounts over years, could add to the harmful effects of cigarettes in this respect. However, in individual cases it is nearly always impossible to attribute such disease to factors other than smoking. Restrictive disease, with reduced vital capacity as well as FEV_1, however, is often more easily attributed to occupational causes, as smoking does not lead to this pattern of dysfunction.

Reduced lung volumes and transfer factor for carbon monoxide are the physiological manifestations of pulmonary fibrosis. Table 2.7 shows the main occupational causes of pulmonary fibrosis and of the acinar inflammation that leads to it.

Asbestosis is a progressive disease in which lower zone fibrosis gradually spreads up the lungs. It occurs in people with prolonged and heavy exposure to asbestos (ship repair, insulation, building work, asbestos textiles) and may sometimes present after exposure has ceased. Almost half of all victims eventually develop lung cancer also.

Silicosis is also progressive. It presents with asymptomatic nodules in the upper zones which become more profuse and enlarge. Eventually they

Table 2.7 Occupational syndromes of fibrosis

Cause	Clinical features	Radiograph
Asbestos	Breathlessness, clubbing, basal crackles	Progressive lower zone fibrosis, pleural plaques
Quartz, Coal dust	Breathlessness, No physical signs	Nodular lesions with conglomeration into large masses. Progressive change
Beryllium	Breathlessness, basal crackles, responds to steroids	Diffuse, irregular fibrosis
Mouldy hay dust (thermophilic actinomycetes)	Often history of previous acute attacks. chronic breathlessness, basal crackles. Partial response to steroids	Upper lobe fibrosis

conglomerate into large masses, causing a mixed restrictive and obstructive pattern of lung function. Miners, stonemasons and quarrymen, tunnellers and fettlers are at risk if exposed to quartz (crystalline silicon dioxide). Rapidly progressive acute and accelerated forms may occur in response to massive exposures.

Berylliosis is a granulomatous Type 4 immunological reaction to inhaled beryllium fume, mainly in refining and occasionally in electronics and the nuclear industry. It may mimic sarcoidosis, causing diffuse irregular fibrosis, but unlike other pneumoconioses responds partially to steroids.

No symptoms, but abnormal chest film

Some occupational lung diseases cause abnormalities of the chest radiograph but no associated symptoms or functional abnormality. Pleural plaques, which often calcify, may be quite extensive as a result of asbestos exposure, and when they are found on a routine film cause the patient a lot of anxiety. They are harmless, the only potential future problems being related to the level of exposure to asbestos and not to the presence of plaques. Coalworkers' pneumoconiosis also may cause a heavy profusion of spots on the film without any functional impairment. Here the risk is of future development of massive fibrosis, a risk related to the profusion of small nodules. However, if a miner has no massive fibrosis, any symptoms should not be attributed to the pneumoconiosis.

Case history 2.7

A 60 year-old coalminer presented to his doctor with increasing shortness of breath over 2 years. He had never smoked, but had extensive nodular shadowing on his chest film. The radiologist reported category 3 simple pneumoconiosis. His doctor told him he was suffering from dust on his lungs and that nothing could be done. The specialist took a more detailed history, noted the initial episodic nature of the breathlessness and the important feature of nocturnal attacks, found him to have severe airflow obstruction and diagnosed asthma. His symptoms were relieved completely by bronchodilators and inhaled steroids. His pneumoconiosis remained unchanged.

Other pneumoconioses due to inhalation of tin refining fumes, iron oxide in welding and metal polishing, and barium sulphate in its production cause dramatic X-ray abnormalities and no harm. Note, however, that tin and barium mining and polishing of metal castings may cause silicosis, a progressive and disabling disease.

Chest pain

Two asbestos-related diseases may present with chest pain, usually associated with breathlessness. Mesothelioma is a malignant disease of the pleura (rarely the peritoneum) caused mainly by exposure to crocidolite asbestos in shipyards and insulation work (building, pipe lagging, railway workshops), several decades previously. It causes progressive obliteration of a hemithorax by tumour and effusion, spreads mainly locally within the thorax, and is fatal within a year or two of diagnosis. It occurs in about 700 people annually in Britain. Rarely, acute pleural effusion occurs in asbestos workers. This resolves spontaneously, leaving pleural thickening by fibrosis. Such pleural thickening may also occur without prior effusion and may cause a mild restrictive pattern of lung function, usually without symptoms.

Pneumonia

Case history 2.8

Over the course of 10 years, three men aged between 25 and 35 from one factory were admitted to the local hospital with fulminating bilateral bronchopneumonia. Bacteriological examination of sputum was negative, white cell counts were below 12,000 in each case, and all had high fever. Two had a prior history of diarrhoea and malaise over a one-week period. All were treated with broad spectrum antibiotics, oxygen and ventilatory support, but died of progressive respiratory failure. Post-mortem examination showed the pathology of adult respiratory distress syndrome in their lungs, but bacteriology was again unhelpful. In no case was the workplace suspected as a cause of the disease.

This coincidence was of course more striking to workers and management in the factory, who initiated investigations. The factory produced chemicals by a biotechnological process, using Aspergillus niger. The three men had all worked in the same part of the factory, and all had been doing the same job at the time of the annual shutdown for cleaning and repairs. All had been exposed to aerosols from water sprayed into contaminated areas. Extensive investigations failed to find a bacterial cause, and Legionella was excluded. However, it was concluded that the workplace was the likely source of infection, and appropriate steps were taken to sterilize contaminated areas and protect workers from aerosols in future.

This case illustrates the often forgotten fact that pneumonia is acquired from the environment. With unusual types of pneumonia it is sensible to enquire about the workplace, and especially about the possibility of aerosols of recirculated or contaminated water. The best known cause is Legionnaires' disease, spread by circulation of droplets from contaminated air-conditioners and cooling systems.

The hand, arm and back

Raynaud's syndrome

Case history 2.9

During an investigation of silicosis among stonemasons, four of ten men were found also to complain of their fingers becoming painful and numb in cold weather. The worst affected had had the condition for four years and it involved all the fingers of his right hand. In cold weather they blanched, became numb, and when he warmed them up, became painful. It was difficult for him to do his job, which involved the use of pneumatic chisels on hard sandstone in an open shed exposed to the west wind sweeping over the Scottish Highlands (Fig. 2.8).

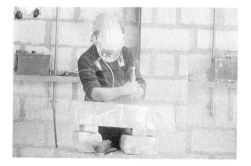

Fig. 2.8 Stonemason working in open with pneumatic powered buffer

This condition is known as vibration white finger, due primarily to vascular spasm induced by using tools vibrating mainly in the range 20-400Hz. It may become a permanent disability even after use of the tools ceases, and any manual worker presenting with the features of Raynaud's disease should be questioned about the use of tools. Occasionally, gangrene of finger tips or permanent loss of finger sensation may occur. Heavy percussive instruments may cause chronic damage to bones and joints in the hands, a different syndrome which may be associated with radiological evidence of bone cysts.

Upper limb strain disorders

Pain on movement of the arm or hands is a very commonly seen syndrome in general practice and orthopaedic clinics. Whether the pain comes from the shoulder (frozen shoulder, rotator cuff syndrome), elbow (tennis elbow, golfers' elbow), forearm (tenosynovitis) or hand (trigger finger, de Quervain's syndrome), the patient's occupation may be an aetiological factor. In such cases, details of the work performed must always be sought. Frequently repetitive movements, often in awkward positions of the joints, are the usual cause. People most at risk are keyboard and visual display unit operators, assembly line workers, hairdressers, cleaners, musicians and music teachers. Carpal tunnel syndrome, typically presenting with paraesthesiae in the median nerve distribution, may also occur as a response to repeated pressure on the palmar aspect of the hand and wrist at work.

While such conditions are very common, according to the Labour Force Survey afflicting up to 60,000 people in the UK, the cause is often missed. They may then become chronic and eventually the sufferer will be unable to continue in the job. On the other hand, if they are diagnosed early, steps can usually be taken to redesign or modify the tasks and the condition may then remit (and be prevented in others). Most of these syndromes may be prevented by proper ergonomic design of jobs (see Chapter 5).

The painful back

It is likely that most orthopaedic conditions related to wear and tear are contributed to by heavy physical work. The most problematical of these from an occupational point of view are those causing low back pain. It is important to recognize two syndromes, the management of which is discussed in Chapters 4 and 8. First, acute disc prolapse which is usually provoked by a sudden strain on the lumbar spine and which is associated with sciatic pain, limitation of spinal flexion and straight leg raising and, often, neurological signs. This condition occurs frequently as a result of awkward lifting or sudden back strains in the workplace and is a major cause of loss of work. In a large hospital, as many as one nurse every week may be expected to present with an acute back injury caused by lifting or catching a patient. The incidence of the condition may be reduced by proper design of the workplace and of the tasks, provision of appropriate aids and training in lifting techniques.

The other syndrome is the chronically painful back with limitation of movement, usually occurring in older male workers, and associated with degenerative changes in the spinal joints. Sometimes pain in the legs on walking and evidence of nerve root compression indicate stenosis of the spinal canal and compression of nerves as they pass out through the neural foramina. It is likely that this condition, which progressively disables people from physical work, is largely contributed to by repeated trauma to the back.

Apart from these two conditions, both of which have at least the potential to be alleviated surgically, there are many other syndromes of back pain which are seen frequently in occupational medical practice. Most commonly, patients present with lumbar ache, usually associated with uncomfortable postures or repeated bending and twisting. Similar complaints are often related to the neck and thoracic spine. Other patients complain of stiffness or lack of mobility, impairing their ability to perform their job. These syndromes have in common a lack of physical signs and a tendency to improve with rest. In all, redesign of the job will be more likely to alleviate the condition than the attentions of an orthopaedic surgeon.

Back problems are important in occupational medicine for two reasons. First, care in the design of the job can play a large part in preventing them and, second, they are responsible for a considerable amount of sickness absence, afflicting about 500,000 people currently in the UK.

The hip

Osteoarthritis of the hip, a very common condition in the elderly, may be contributed to by occupational factors. Workers such as farmers, who spend much of their lives in physical activity, have an increased risk of this disease.

The ear

Hearing loss and tinnitus

The first symptom of noise-induced hearing loss is usually difficulty hearing a conversation against a noisy background. The patient comes to dislike parties where everyone is apparently chattering away happily, yet he or she hears just a jumble of noise. Consonants seem to be lost first. Often the patients will mention intermittent high-pitched ringing in the ears, though this is rarely sufficient to be more than an irritant. By the time these symptoms have become sufficient to force medical consultation, the damage as measured by audiometry will be severe and, even with cessation of noise exposure, progressive.

Workers at special risk of hearing damage are usually those in heavy productive industry, such as metal work, drilling and quarrying, stone cutting, or the use of noisy machinery, as in textiles, printing, wood cutting, transportation and agriculture. Noises above 90 dB, as measured with special instruments that are electronically weighted to mimic loudness functions of the human ear, are likely to cause damage to a proportion of the exposed population with continued exposure. Very high levels may cause damage after relatively short periods, even when the noise is intermittent. This may be illustrated by the frequent finding of hearing loss in people who have fired guns as an occasional hobby, as well as in people who are exposed to noise of lower levels but more constantly, such as those working on construction sites.

High noise levels damage the hair cells of the organ of Corti, affecting first those in the basal part of the cochlea concerned with reception of the highest frequency sounds and progressing through to those receiving lower frequencies. This is reflected in audiometric changes which show loss of sound perception first in the 4-5 kilohertz (kHz) range, progressing both in severity and into lower frequency ranges (Fig 2.9). When hearing is reduced at 3kHz and below, conversation is interfered with.

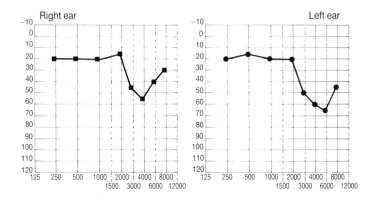

Fig. 2.9   Bilateral noise-induced hearing loss in audiogram of a papermill worker

The harmful effects of noise are cumulative and not, of course, confined to the workplace. The use of personal stereos and frequenting of discos has resulted in young people having some early damage to hearing before they even start work. As well as attempting to protect workers from noise, many companies now carry out pre-employment audiometry.

The eye

Sore eyes

Complaints about sore or aching eyes are among the most common symptoms encountered by occupational physicians in organizations which use visual display units. They are rarely serious or even accompanied by evidence of a defect of refraction, but usually indicate poor design of the workplace, in terms of lighting, screen reflectance or even posture at the desk. In contrast, eye injury due to foreign body or burns is potentially very serious and is a common, though easily preventable, problem in manufacturing industry.

Eye injury may also occur as a result of exposure to light – keratitis is conjunctivitis caused by inadequate eye protection in arc welding, while accidental exposure of the eye to laser beams (sometimes reflected inadvertently off a polished surface) may cause serious corneal or retinal burns. Protection from lasers depends critically on the wavelength of the light, and goggles must be specific to the laser being used.

Itchy eyes

Itchy eyes are a frequent complaint in workers exposed to organic antigen, such as animal dander and grain dusts. This symptom is often a herald of occupational asthma. Non-allergic eye irritation by, for example, chlorine or formaldehyde, is also a common complaint.

The nose

Rhinitis

Allergic rhinitis is a common herald of occupational asthma, usually in association with exposure to organic antigen from vegetable matter or from animals, and it is not uncommon to see patients in whom the rhinitis is the sole manifestation of such allergy. Nasal polyposis may occur in severe cases.

Septal ulceration

Ulceration of the nasal septum, often painless, has been described following uncontrolled exposures to metal fume or dust; chromates (sometimes in cement) are the best known cause, though in earlier times arsenic and mercury were recognized causes.

Carcinoma

Carcinoma of the nasal sinuses has been described as a consequence of exposure to dust in furniture and leather goods manufacture, where the rare adenocarcinoma seems to be the usual histological type. Nasal carcinomas have also occurred following exposure to nickel subsulphide and bischloromethyl ether.

The nervous system

Case history 2.10

A 58 year-old man presented to a neurologist with muscular weakness and unsteadiness, affecting mainly his legs and fine movements of his hands. The condition had developed insidiously over about four years, but had been brought to medical attention when he was referred to an occupational physician as being suspected of drunkenness at work. The physician found that he was a teetotaller, but that he had bilateral brisk reflexes and some hand-nose incoordination. The neurologist found signs of neurological disease affecting cerebellar and pyramidal tracts, with no sensory involvement. Routine tests, including CT scan, were unhelpful but electromyograms showed some evidence of denervation. No firm diagnosis was made, but arrangements were made to follow him up and assess the progress of the condition.

The patient himself wondered if his work was responsible and, after consulting his trade union, took a civil action against his employer. His work had involved 12 years of painting within the hulls of ships, often in very confined spaces. He had always used spray paints, solvent-based but of several different sorts. He had never used respiratory protection and had done paint spraying for at least four hours every day, five days per week.

His illness forced him to retire from work. Over the course of the next 18 months he showed a slow improvement in his ability to perform physical tasks. Review by the neurologist confirmed that a previously progressive condition had ceased to deteriorate, but that the pattern of symptoms and signs did not fit with any recognized neurological syndrome. Further investigation showed that, of the patient's eight colleagues in the dockyard paint shop, one had died with cerebellar degeneration and respiratory failure and two others had serious neurological disease.

Very many workers in Britain are exposed to solvents, chemicals that by their nature are themselves lipid-soluble and therefore capable of retention in nervous tissue. Painting, cleaning, carpet-tile laying, laboratory and chemical work, degreasing operations and exposure to petroleum are just a few of the situations in which high exposures may occur. Moreover, exposure in hobbies such as model making or DIY, may add to that at work. Solvent exposure may also occur as a form of substance abuse – the best known types being alcoholism and glue-sniffing.

Physicians should be alert to the possibility of solvent exposure contributing to or causing neuro-psychiatric disease. This ranges from a syndrome of headache, loss of concentration and short-term memory, and depression to full-blown dementia or neurological disease such as peripheral neuropathy, cerebellar ataxia or motor neurone disease. In particular, if the presentation is in any way clinically unusual or atypical of the well-known syndromes of neurological disease, the possibility of occupational causation should be borne in mind.

Peripheral neuropathy

A motor neuropathy, characteristically with wrist drop, is a classical feature of lead poisoning, now rarely seen. Mixed sensorimotor neuropathy may occur after exposure to acrylamide, n-hexane, methyl butyl ketone and some mercury compounds.

Parkinsonism

Chronic manganese poisoning, prolonged exposure to carbon disulphide and acute carbon monoxide poisoning may all lead to the development of a Parkinsonian syndrome, as well as to other central nervous system damage.

Other neurological syndromes

A wide range of syndromes has been described in relation to occupational exposures. Some are shown in Table 2.8.

Table 2.8   Some neurotoxic effects of occupational exposures

Syndrome	Toxic agents	Occupations
Narcosis	Solvents, vinyl chloride	Degreasing, tank cleaning
Organic psychosis	Carbon disulphide mercury	Viscose rayon manufacture Pressure measurement
Behavioural disorders	Solvents Styrene	Painting, degreasing Polymerisation
Pyramidal tract disease	Solvents	Painting, degreasing
Parkinsonism	Carbon disulphide Carbon monoxide Manganese	Viscose rayon manufacture Exposure to fire Battery, alloy work
Cerebellar disease	Alcohol Solvents	Bar work Painting, degreasing
Diffuse neurological disease	Gas embolism	Diving, caisson work
Autonomic hyperactivity	Anticholinesterase pesticides	Horticulture, agriculture
Bladder neuropathy	Dimethylaminopropionitrile	Polyurethane manufacture
Peripheral neuropathy	Lead Acrylamide Hexane, methyl butyl ketone	Smelting Polymerisation Solvent use, degreasing

Stress reactions

The majority of patients seen in occupational medical practice with neuropsychiatric symptoms are suffering psychological rather than chemical stress. Such patients commonly present with a picture of anxiety and depression, and an array of minor physical symptoms. A history of adverse reaction to stress at previous times is often present, and the causes are usually multiple involving home and family as well as work. Women with two jobs, one at home and one at work, are particularly vulnerable, especially when their jobs, as is often the case, are poorly paid and offer little prospect of satisfaction or promotion. People promoted beyond their capabilities or switched to new technology are also at risk. Some factors in the workplace to look out for are shown in Table 2.9.

Table 2.9 Common adverse factors in the workplace leading to psychological breakdown

---

Recent promotion beyond capacity
Conflicts due to multiple responsibilities
Too many demands on time
A tiring shift pattern, excess overtime
Too little or boring work
New technology
A new or unreasonable boss
Increased productivity targets
Threat of redundancy
Sexual harassment or bullying
High sickness absence in colleagues

Personal factors are of course important, some people thriving on what would grind others into the ground. Physical ill health is often the last straw in an otherwise marginally adjusted individual.

Psychological problems, often of a relatively minor nature, are commonplace in occupational health practice, usually presenting through management referral for repeated or prolonged sickness absence. The spectrum of these conditions is wide, from frankly psychotic illness, through serious depression with suicide risk to mild anxiety and simple dislike of work. Assessment of provocative workplace factors, potentially amenable to intervention, requires time and patience, especially when (as is often the case) the patient presents with somatic symptoms.

Case history 2.11

A 55 year-old consultant community physician was referred to occupational health because of prolonged sickness absence. He was severely depressed and somewhat hostile, suspecting (probably rightly) that the referral was motivated by a desire to terminate his employment on grounds of ill-health. Some personal and domestic factors were put forward as explanation of his mood change, but changes at work connected with Health Service reorganization had been dramatic. These had involved a considerable increase in work-load, the introduction of unrealistic targets and the expectation that he would always take work home with him. Pressures of the same nature on his superiors were being passed down and there was little sympathy in the department for those who were unable to keep up.

After a series of discussions with the patient, his general practitioner and (respecting medical confidentiality) his superior, it proved possible to plan a course of rehabilitation to work which took account of the patient's illness and likely response to various stresses in the workplace, and of the effects of the patient's drug therapy.

This case had a moderately successful outcome, as it was possible to modify the patient's workload and to persuade his seniors to be a little more tolerant of someone who clearly had a rather difficult personality. Such cases are often complicated by alcohol abuse and marital difficulties, and management is correspondingly less easy or successful. Nevertheless, clinical skills in eliciting the various provocative factors leading to breakdown are the key to successful intervention. Further discussion of the management of such problems is to be found in Chapters 4 and 7.

Disease of the liver and gastro-intestinal tract

A wide range of liver diseases have occupational causes, but all are rare. In contrast, the gastro-intestinal tract is almost untouched by occupational disease, although oesophageal and stomach cancers occur to excess in rubber vulcanizers and coalminers respectively.

The liver has a key role in transformation of lipid-soluble chemicals into water-soluble ones. While this usually results in a less toxic metabolite, occasionally the reverse occurs. The classic example is acute hepatic necrosis caused by carbon tetrachloride, a condition that used to occur in dry cleaning workers, where free radical formation causes peroxidation of cell membrane lipids. Polychlorinated biphenyls may cause a similar syndrome, and both chemicals may also lead to cirrhosis. Cholestasis has been described following exposure to methylene dianiline in the use of epoxy resins, and portal cirrhosis and haemangiosarcoma may occur as a result of exposure to high levels of vinyl chloride monomer in PVC production. However, even in a worker in the chemical industry, abnormalities of liver function are more likely to be related to alcohol or other causes than to occupational factors.

Urinary tract diseases

Acute renal failure may occur following high level exposure to cadmium dust or fumes by cutting metal alloys, making pigments or battery manufacture. Mercury exposure in, for example, barometer repair or accidental spillage and vaporization of the metal, and carbon tetrachloride exposure may also cause this syndrome. These agents, carbon disulphide and a wide range of solvents may also cause damage to the nephron and chronic renal failure. Bladder cancer has been a well-authenticated risk in workers in the rubber tyre industry and in the manufacture of organic dyes. Benzidine and 2-naphthylamine are the chemicals that have been shown to have this effect, being converted in the liver into carcinogens that then exert their effect on the bladder through excretion in the urine.

Disorders of the reproductive system

Infertility, miscarriage and fetal abnormality may sometimes be blamed on factors at work, and the gynaecologist should always take such a possibility seriously. There is some evidence that heavy physical work during pregnancy may have a harmful effect on the outcome, and there are plenty of opportunities during the process of gametogenesis, fertilization and pregnancy for toxic substances to exert an effect. The effects of ionizing radiation are well known, as are those of handling cytotoxic drugs. Less well known are the effects of chlorinated biphenyls on microsomal enzymes in the liver, increasing their ability to metabolize oral contraceptives and thus cause pill failure, or the adverse effects on male fertility of work in oestrogen production or of handling dibromochloropropane in nematocide manufacture. Lead, in males and females, and organic mercury in females are potent reproductive poisons, causing infertility, miscarriage and fetal abnormality. Solvents used in the manufacture of electrical and electronic apparatus, and ethylene oxide used in sterilization procedures have also been shown to increase risks of miscarriage. However, suggestions that anaesthetic gases, in levels normally found in operating theatres. and non-ionizing radiation from visual display units are harmful have not been supported by scientific investigation.

Blood disorders

While all are rare, toxic effects of workplace substances may cause a wide range of haematological disorders. These are shown in Table 2.10.

In spite of careful regulation, episodes of lead poisoning still occur in industry. The classical features of abdominal colic, motor nerve paralysis and anaemia are fortunately rare, but evidence of excessive exposure in terms of blood levels over 40 μg/100 ml are not infrequent. Above this level inhibition of haem synthesis, related to inhibition of δaminolaevulinic acid dehydratase (δALA-D) and ferrochelatase, may be expected and some interference with central or peripheral nervous function may occur. Reproductive hazards have already been mentioned.

Adverse effects of chronic benzene and radiation exposure have largely been prevented by regulation. Arsine poisoning does however occur sporadically. This gas (hydrogen arsenide) is used in the microelectronics industry, where it is usually handled with great care. It is also given off inadvertently

Table 2.10   Occupational blood disorders

Disorder	Features	Causes
Marrow aplasia	Normocytic anaemia neutropoenia	Benzene, gamma radiation
Anaemia	Impaired haem synthesis stippled red cells	Lead
Methaemoglobinaemia	Cyanosis reversed by methylene blue	Aniline and some of its analogues, nitrites
Haemolysis	Intravascular haemolysis haemoglobinuria	Arsine, trimellitic anhydride
Leukaemia	Usually chronic myeloid occasionally acute	Gamma radiation, benzene
Thrombocytopoenia	Bleeding disorder	Toluene diisocyanate

when metal containing traces of arsenic is burnt or treated with acid, or when hot metal is cooled with water. Cases occur in the scrap metal industry.

Cardiac disease

There is strong evidence of association between risk of heart disease and specific occupation in three circumstances: workers exposed to carbon disulphide in manufacture of viscose rayon have an increased likelihood of death from coronary artery disease; people exposed to nitrates such as glyceryl trinitrate and ethylene glycol dinitrate in manufacture of explosives and of pharmaceuticals have an increased risk of angina and infarction; and those exposed to high levels of halogenated organic solvents such as trichloroethylene may suffer sudden death, probably related to ventricular fibrillation. Carbon monoxide exposures of the levels to which some workers may be subjected in industry probably do not reach those generated by cigarette smoking, and have not been shown convincingly to increase risk of heart attack.

General ill-health and infection

The most difficult patients to investigate and manage in medical practice are often those with non-specific symptoms of malaise and general ill-health. As with all other symptom complexes, the occupational history may lead to diagnosis and appropriate management. The most important occupational factors are psychological problems and physical problems associated with the building in which the person works, the two not infrequently interacting. Less commonly, chronic poisoning or occupational infection may occur.

Case history 2.12

A 38 year-old lady presented with complaints of tiredness, headaches and blurred vision, which she attributed to the use of a visual display unit (VDU) in a hospital switchboard. There were no physical abnormalities and testing of her vision was normal. Inspection of the workplace showed good ergonomic design of the workstation, appropriate positioning and anti-reflective screening of the VDU, and adequate temperature and humidity control of the room. Further investigation, however, showed a high sickness absence rate among the operators, many complaints of bad temperature control and general dissatisfaction with the job. An alcohol problem was found in one operator and a long-term health problem in another, leading to a requirement on the others to do excessive overtime. In addition, the staff were all women who combined their jobs with domestic responsibilities. The patient herself had worked seven days a week for three weeks!

Almost everyone in that workplace had symptoms related to the pressures of the job. They were relieved when the long-term problems were dealt with, extra staff were taken on and overtime reduced. The temperature complaints were solved by asking the staff to decide on what temperature they preferred, and setting it at that.

This history illustrates one of the many ways in which workplace stress may present with somatic symptoms. Often the full story only comes out when the workplace is visited, giving the occupational physician an advantage over the general practitioner.

Vague physical symptoms occur not infrequently in workers in modern buildings, especially those built to conserve energy with recirculating air and in which individuals have little or no control over their environment. The symptoms include headaches, pain in the face, sore or dry throats, loss of voice, wheeziness, cough and general malaise. They are typically better at weekends and on holiday. Sometimes investigation of the building shows a contaminated air-conditioning system, spreading amoebal antigen and Gram-negative bacterial endotoxin around the building. Often, however, nothing is found other than recirculated air and windows that do not open. This condition has acquired the inapt name of the 'sick building syndrome', but is better called 'building related sickness'.

Case history 2.13

Several radiographers reported cough and wheeze when working in their department, which was situated in a basement and ventilated artificially. Investigation of the workforce showed widespread complaints of malaise, itchy skins, sore eyes, cough and, in two dramatic cases, loss of voice within an hour of entering the department. The air conditioning system was uncontaminated and the temperature and humidity control adequate (excessive dryness is an important cause of itchy skins in workplaces). However, the ceiling tiles were perforated and covered with loose glass wool. These tiles were regularly being disturbed by building work. When the glass wool was removed and replaced by insulation in bags all the complaints ceased, suggesting strongly that they had been due to an irritant reaction to the mineral fibres.

Occupational infections may sometimes be severe, as when *Legionella sp* contaminate an air conditioner and cause outbreaks of pneumonia or when a farmer is infected by *Leptospira sp* and dies of hepato-renal failure. Occasionally chronic debilitating infections cause diagnostic problems – the two best known are infection by *Brucella sp*, a hazard of farmers and veterinary surgeons, and Lyme disease, caused by *Borrelia burgdorferi* infection acquired by a tick bite in deer country and therefore a hazard of forestry workers. This latter condition often starts with a spreading erythematous lesion at the site of the bite (usually the lower leg), accompanied by influenza-like symptoms and enlarged lymph nodes. Subsequently the patient may develop meningitis and radiculopathies, polyarthritis and myopericarditis. These manifestations are very variable and may occur up to two years after initial infection. Transmission of the bacterium across the placenta may cause abortion or fetal abnormality. Early diagnosis, achieved by suspecting the disease in those exposed to deer country, and antibiotic treatment is very important.

Chronic poisoning in the workplace is relatively uncommon in the developed world, although episodes of lead and mercury poisoning still occur. More commonly, recurrent overdosage with pesticides and solvents may be seen, often leading to non-specific symptoms. Farmers and fruit growers may easily spray themselves with carbamate or organophosphorous insecticides and manifest symptoms of anticholinesterase poisoning – headache, blurred vision, weakness, sweating and tremor. Recurrent exposure to solvents is particularly liable to occur in the self-employed or in people employed in small companies involving painting and floor covering with flexible vinyl materials. Headaches and a feeling of drunkenness are the usual features, with the threat of long-term neurological damage.

3

Investigation of occupational disease

Summary

In the investigation of occupational disease, there are three complementary methods. The clinical approach uses history, examination and special tests to reach a diagnosis of disease and cause. This is often sufficient for the patient's purposes, so long as the cause may be avoided in the future. However, the clinical approach does not take account of the need to eliminate the cause in order to prevent similar disease in others. For this, a visit to the workplace is necessary. This is best done by someone, such as an occupational physician, who is familiar with the methods. Full investigation of a workplace may require some knowledge of occupational hygiene, toxicology and ergonomics. The objective of a workplace investigation is to find hazards and reduce the risks from them, and this chapter describes means of making such an investigation.

The third approach is the epidemiological, which may be used to investigate possible causes of disease or their effects, to measure risks from exposure to harmful environments or substances and to test the effectiveness of preventive measures. In designing an epidemiological study many practical matters need to be considered, such as time, costs, validity of tests, and methods of selecting, sampling and ensuring attendance; great care has to be taken to design a study appropriate to the hypothesis to be tested, and the main types of such study are explained. Finally, two notes of caution are given with respect to problems arising from screening for disease and jumping too readily to conclusions about environmental factors and disease causation.

Introduction

Doctors may encounter great difficulty in investigating occupational disease. Consider the following case history:

Case history 3.1

A 40 year-old man had developed progressive shortness of breath over 12 months. There were no physical signs of respiratory disease other than breathlessness at rest, and a chest film showed diffuse hazy shadowing in both lungs with some irregular fibrosis in the upper zones. Lung function showed a severe restrictive pattern with gas transfer reduced to 30 per cent of the predicted value.

He had been a stone mason for 24 years, and for the last four had been working on a mediaeval cathedral, renovating the window tracery with newly quarried sandstone, and using pneumatic chisels and saws. The physician made a diagnosis of silicosis and referred the patient to the Department of Social Security doctors of the Pneumoconiosis Panel for consideration of compensation. These doctors disagreed with the diagnosis, saying that the X-ray appearances were inconsistent with silicosis.

There was therefore a conflict of opinion. Does the patient have silicosis or some other disease? How may this be resolved? The immediate reaction of the doctor is the clinical approach – to carry out further diagnostic tests.

It was decided to carry out open lung biopsy. The surgeon commented on a nodular feel to the lungs and removed two pieces, one from a part that felt fibrosed and one from a more normal area. The pathologist reported diffuse interstitial fibrosis with desquamation of alveolar cells and no nodular change. Relatively little doubly refractile material was seen and it was concluded that the changes were not due to silicosis but to cryptogenic fibrosis. The patient did not improve with steroid treatment and died of respiratory failure a year later. The death certificate recorded cryptogenic pulmonary fibrosis.

At this stage the physician has accepted what seemed to be expert opinion, although he remained uncertain, since the radiological appearances were quite unlike those of cryptogenic pulmonary fibrosis. Is there any other step that you would have taken at this stage? Unfortunately a necropsy was not carried out when the patient died at home.

Two years later, a second mason from the same workplace presented to the consultant chest physician with similar symptoms and X-ray changes. Again, compensation was refused on the grounds of inconsistent X-ray appearances. On this occasion, an urgent visit to the workplace was arranged (Fig. 3.1). The stone masons were found to be working in primitive conditions, respirable quartz dust levels often reaching 100 times the 8-hour exposure limit. The diagnosis of accelerated silicosis was made and review of the first patient's lung biopsies showed them to contain massive amounts of quartz, generally of particle size too small to show up with polarized light. An epidemiological survey of all 350 masons employed by the same company was arranged and discovered four other men with less severe stages of silicosis.

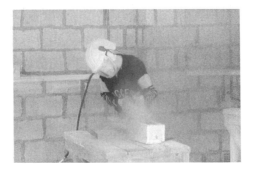

Fig. 3.1 Stonemason generating cloud of quartz dust in cutting sandstone

This episode illustrates the three complementary methods used in the investigation of occupational disease – clinical, workplace and epidemiological. A clinician often finds difficulty with workplace and epidemiological investigation, and it is with these that this chapter is particularly concerned.

Strategy of investigation

The starting point of investigation is the realization by a doctor that the patient may have an occupational disease. This leads to a more detailed occupational history, as described in Chapter 1, and this in itself may be sufficient to confirm the diagnosis. More usually, however, other tests may be necessary – for example, serial measurements of peak flow rate in occupational asthma, audiograms in hearing loss or patch testing in dermatitis. This is the clinical investigation. If an occupational cause seems likely, the clinician is then faced with a two-fold problem. First, the patient may not be able to return to work unless the workplace is modified and, second, if the patient does have an occupational disease, there may well be others in the same workplace exposed to the same risk; some may already have the same disease. Thus, some form of workplace investigation becomes mandatory, perhaps allied to an epidemiological study of the exposed workforce. In this respect, the doctor's role becomes wider than that of simply diagnosing and treating a patient; there is an obligation also to take on a preventive role.

The clinical investigation

The most important component of this is a careful occupational history, as detailed in Chapter 1. Thereafter, investigation depends on the type of disease and the organ or systems affected. The aims of investigation are first to establish the pathological and functional diagnosis and, second, to establish the cause. The former step will only be briefly alluded to here. The latter may require more than clinical skills, and may involve workplace and epidemiological investigation. This is not to say clinical skills are unimportant in occupational practice – on the contrary, they are an essential foundation on which to build, and lack of such skills can be very much to the patient's disadvantage.

Case history 3.2

A general practitioner was employed on a sessional basis at a local chemical factory. As part of his duties, he was asked to make an annual health examination of workers exposed to formaldehyde. One such worker consulted him in his role as general practitioner with symptoms of asthma. The doctor prescribed treatment and, since he had seen him in the surgery, excused him from attending his workplace check-up. The asthma got progressively worse and the patient eventually asked for a second opinion. The consultant confirmed the diagnosis of formaldehyde asthma, but by this time the patient's illness had become severe and persistent, causing him to have to retire on the grounds of ill health. The doctor was sued for negligence.

This case illustrates the dangers of practising in a field of medicine in which you have no training, and also shows what may happen if basic clinical history-taking skills are neglected. Another point, to which we shall return later in this chapter and in Chapter 5, concerns the rationale for screening or 'routine' surveillance. The objectives of such procedures must be clear, as must the action to be taken on finding a positive result.

Skin diseases

Of the conditions mentioned in Chapter 2, contact dermatitis is far and away the most common. The diagnosis of all these conditions depends mainly on a careful history and clinical examination, and often also on obtaining samples of the materials to which the patient has been exposed.

The site of the lesion is of primary importance, though it should be remembered that allergic contact dermatitis may spread to other parts of the body, especially the eyelids. The condition may also be mimicked by non-occupational dermatitis, for example to nickel, spreading to the hands. The time course of the condition and its development in relation to exposure to possible allergens or irritants are also essential details to obtain.

Case history 3.3

A 30 year-old woman started work as a research assistant. She had known for several years that she could not wear cheap jewellery or watches because of the itchy rash they caused. Part of her work involved embedding tissue for sectioning for electron microscopy, using epoxy resin. After a month she noticed itchy hands and a rash on her fingers. Her hands showed an erythematous reaction with tiny vesicles. In addition there was evidence of a reaction under her wedding ring. A clinical diagnosis of nickel and epoxy dermatitis was made and she responded to a change of work practice avoiding contact with epoxy resin. Subsequent patch testing confirmed the diagnosis.

The usual problem in occupational skin disease is differentiation of allergic and irritant contact dermatitis (Table 3.1). For this, the use of patch testing is often essential.

Table 3.1   Clues to differentiating allergic and irritant dermatitis*

	Irritant	Allergic
Common causes	Detergents, cleaning materials, oils, dusts	Low molecular weight chemicals (cobalt, nickel, colophony, epoxy resins, formaldehyde)
Onset	May be acute or subacute	Days or weeks after exposure
Distribution	Backs of hands then palms	Site of contact, plus eyelids frequently
Progression	Tendency to local worsening	Spreads to other parts of skin
Patch tests	Negative	Positive

Note: It is often not possible to differentiate the two conditions clinically

Patch testing

Patch tests are used to diagnose allergic contact dermatitis. The suspected antigens, or more commonly a battery of antigens including those suspected, are placed on absorbent material in small aluminium strips or chambers and applied by permeable tape to an area of unaffected skin, usually the back (Fig. 3.2). They are left in place for 48 hours, removed and then inspected for evidence of a reaction about 30 minutes later, and then at intervals over the next week. Care is necessary to avoid using irritant concentrations of chemicals, which may give a spuriously positive result. A true allergic reaction usually shows erythema and induration, but vesiculation and blistering may occur in severe ones. The reaction, being one of delayed hypersensitivity, may occur up to five days after application of the antigen. It typically increases in size and severity over a few days, and this is one feature that helps distinguish it from an irritant dermatitis (Table 3.2).

The choice of antigen for patch testing depends on the suspected cause. One battery commonly used and available commercially is given in Table 3.3.

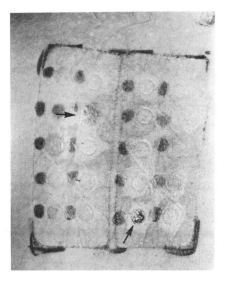

Fig. 3.2 Patch testing on a nurse with allergy to surgical gloves. Positive results to thiuram mix (upper arrow) and nickel sulphate (lower arrow)

Table 3.2 Differentiating irritant and allergic dermatitis on patch testing

Irritant	Allergic
High concentrations	Reaction occurs with low concentrations
Affects most people exposed	Substance affects relatively few individuals
Reaction comes and goes quickly	Develops late and gets worse

Table 3.3 Useful occupational contact dermatitis patch tests

Sensitizer	Some sources in workplaces
Potassium dichromate	Cement, paints, tanning
Cobalt chloride	Cement, coolant oils
Nickel sulphate	Plating, use of tools
Colophony	Glues, solder flux, adhesive plaster
Wool alcohols	Handling woollens
Formaldehyde	Disinfectants
Thiurams	Rubber, adhesives, pesticides
Mercaptones	Rubber
Mercaptobenzthiazoles	Rubber
Paraphenylene diamine	Dyes, hairdressing
Epoxy resins	Adhesives, paints
Primin	Primulas

Other diagnostic aids

Occasionally skin biopsy and appropriate staining may be necessary to make a diagnosis in obscure cases of occupational skin disease. In patients exposed to hydroquinone and p-tertiary butylphenol at risk of vitiligo, a Wood's lamp may be helpful for medical surveillance and detection of early cases.

Lung diseases

As with skin disease, the diagnosis of occupational lung disease depends critically on a history that takes account of the development and evolution of symptoms in relation to exposure to suspected causes. In contrast, physical examination is much less useful and the diagnosis is usually clinched by relatively simple investigations. Some conditions may not be diagnosed with the usually accepted degree of clinical confidence – for example, it is rarely possible to be sure that emphysema or lung cancer are occupational in aetiology. The most useful tests are described briefly below.

Chest radiography

The main use of radiography is in the diagnosis of the pneumoconioses, and a classification of typical appearances is given in the Fig. 3.3. Amorphous particles, such as quartz and coal cause small discrete nodular lesions that may aggregate together to form large masses (known as PMF or progressive massive fibrosis). Asbestos causes diffuse fine irregular shadows, predominantly in lower zones. Berylliosis causes coarser irregular shadows throughout the lungs, while chronic allergic alveolitis may cause irregular streaky shadows in the upper zones. Appearances mimicking cardiac pulmonary oedema may occur in acute allergic alveolitis and toxic pneumonitis.

Lung function testing

Lung function tests measure the pathophysiological effects of the disease, and are therefore usually only complementary to other procedures in reaching a diagnosis. The main changes found in occupational lung diseases are given in Table 3.4 – note the important negative findings in simple pneumoconiosis.

The most useful tests in a diagnostic sense are those used in monitoring changes, in relation either to exposure in the workplace or challenge testing.

Disease	Radiograph	Differential diagnosis
Simple pneumoconiosis (coal, silica, mixed dust, etc.)		Multiple matastases Miliary tuberculosis Sarcoidosis
Progressive massive fibrosis (coal, silica)		Primary & secondary cancer Tuberculosis Lung abscess
Mesothelioma (asbestos)		Pleural effusion (other causes) Pleural metastases Pleural fibrosis
Acute allergic alveolitis		Pulmonary oedema Pulmonary eosinophilia Sarcoidosis Atypical pneumonia
Chronic allergic alveolitis		Healed tuberculosis Chronic sarcoidosis Ankylosing spondylitis lung
Berylliosis		Chronic sarcoidosis Cystic fibrosis
Asbestosis Aluminium lung		Cryptogenic fibrosis
Pleural plaques and fibrosis (asbestos)		Pleural fat deposits

Fig. 3.3 Classification used in the radiographic diagnosis of pneumoconioses

Table 3.4   Functional changes in occupational lung diseases

Disease	Changes
Simple pneumoconiosis	Usually none
PMF	Mixed restriction and obstruction
Asbestosis	Restriction and reduced gas transfer
Allergic alveolitis	Reduced gas transfer
Toxic pneumonitis	Reduced gas transfer
Berylliosis	Restriction and reduced gas transfer
Asthma	Variable airflow obstruction

In suspected occupational asthma, it is usual to carry out serial recordings of peak flow rate, the readings being made by the patient several times daily over a month (Fig. 3.4). At least two weeks' recordings should be done when the patient is off work, and the record inspected for differences in level when exposed and not exposed. If clear reduction in flow rates occur while at work, occupational asthma is likely and a sensitizing agent is usually easily identified. If one is not obvious from the history, inspection of the workplace (see later) and subsequent challenge testing may be necessary.

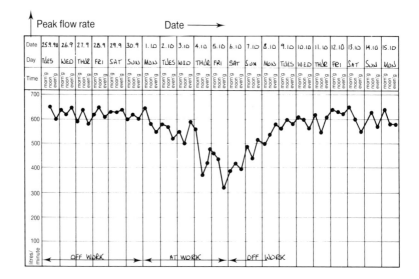

Fig. 3.4   Peak flow rate recorded in a man working unloading grain at an animal foodstuff manufacturer. Note fall in flow rate during period at work

Case history 3.4

A 30 year-old laboratory technician complained of increasingly troublesome asthma, worse while at work and usually starting 2–3 hours after starting each day. He also had noticed attacks of wheeze after drinking red wine, but was otherwise well. His work involved serology in relation to Hepatitis B and HIV diagnosis. Peak flow recordings confirmed substantial falls during the working week and normal values when off work. No known sensitizer was present among the chemicals he used and nothing suspicious was seen on inspection of the laboratory. However, the patient himself wondered if the powder used on his rubber gloves, which he changed repeatedly, might be responsible.

Some of the glove powder (starch) and talc as control were used in challenge tests and produced no response in lung function. However, when he was challenged by putting on and removing rubber gloves he did show a sharp fall in peak flow – but only when using the batch of gloves used in his laboratory. Subsequent testing showed that these gloves, but not the control gloves, gave off a vapour containing the known sensitizer D-carene.

Challenge testing should only be done in a hospital setting, since delayed and severe reactions may occur. This said, it is a relatively simple procedure whereby dilutions of the suspected causative agent are either nebulized or put into the air by tipping from dish to dish or other straightforward manner so that the patient can inhale it and the functional effect can be measured. The closer the challenge mimics the actual workplace exposure, the better (Fig. 3.5).

In asthma, both an immediate and a delayed fall in peak flow may occur,

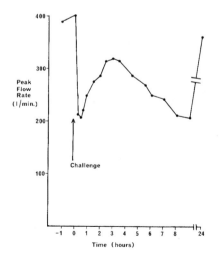

Fig. 3.5 Immediate and delayed responses to challenge testing with isocyanates

the latter lasting up to 48 hours. In allergic alveolitis, the response is a rise in temperature, a feeling of malaise and a fall in gas transfer at about three hours, lasting up to 48 hours.

Other tests

In asthma, positive results to skin prick testing would be expected to protein antigens and to some chemicals such as complex salts of platinum, though not to colophony or isocyanates. This test is done by lifting the epidermis with a fine needle through a drop of antigen. Similarly, positive radio-allergosorbent (RAST) tests may be helpful in diagnosis if an antigen is available. In allergic alveolitis skin tests are not advisable, but precipitating antibodies to the common antigens may be found. These are useful in the presence of disease, but do not of themselves indicate that lung disease is present.

Lung biopsy and study of broncho-alveolar lavage fluid are occasionally helpful in the investigation of obscure cases, usually to differentiate between occupational and non-occupational disease.

Occupational poisonings

A wide variety of syndromes, discussed in Chapter 2, may be caused by occupational exposure to toxic substances. Again, the diagnosis rests largely on the occupational history and an awareness that exposure to gases, fumes and chemicals may lead to disease. In general, toxic gases and fumes attack the lung, metals damage internal organs, solvents cause damage to the nervous system, and a number of insecticides cause symptoms of parasympathetic overactivity. There are some investigations that are of value in establishing a diagnosis and monitoring exposure or response to treatment in some of these poisonings; the more important ones are summarized in Table 3.5.

In general, inorganic chemicals may be measured in either blood or urine, and some (such as mercury and arsenic which accumulate in the tissues) in hair and nail parings. The metabolites of organic substances which are rapidly biotransformed into water-soluble chemicals may be measured in urine, while poorly biotransformed organics are measured in blood. Volatile organics (of which the best known example is ethyl alcohol) may be measured in alveolar air. In cases of suspected chronic poisoning by metals such as lead, mercury or cadmium, *in vivo* methods using neutron activation or X-ray fluorescence are being developed. There is further discussion of biological monitoring in Chapter 5.

Investigation of the workplace

This is the aspect of occupational medicine with which doctors are least familiar. Indeed, almost no doctor thinks to visit a patient's workplace and

Table 3.5   Occupational poisonings

	Poison	Clinical features	Investigations
Metals	Inorganic lead	lethargy and fatigue abdominal pain constipation vomiting rarely, anaemia and neuropathy	blood lead raised urinary δ-amino laevulinic acid raised red cell protoporphyrin
	Organic lead	sleep disturbance nausea anorexia	urine lead
	Mercury acute	fever tremor pneumonitis	blood and urine mercury levels – may be misleading because of irregular excretion
	chronic	gingivitis tremor cerebellar signs psychotic features	
	Cadmium acute	fever pneumonitis renal cortical necrosis	urine cadmium
	chronic	renal tubular dysfunction ?emphysema	urine B_2 microglobulin urine N-acetyl glucosaminidase (nonspecific)
	Beryllium acute	pneumonitis allergic dermatitis	urine beryllium
	chronic	pulmonary fibrosis	lymphocyte transformation and macrophage inhibition tests
Pesticides	Organophosphorus (e.g. parathion)	headache, nausea abdominal pain twitching small pupils convulsions	reduced blood cholinesterase, urine p-nitrophenol
	Carbamates	as organophosphorus	reduced blood cholinesterase,
	Organochlorine (e.g. lindane)	headache abdominal pain ataxia tremor	specific agent in blood
	Pyrethrum	dermatitis	urine pyrethroids

Table 3.5   Occupational poisonings (continued)

	Poison	Clinical features	Investigations
Herbicides	Substituted phenols (e.g. dinitro orthocresol)	hyperpyrexia	blood dinitro orthocresol
	Bipyridyls (e.g. paraquat)	pulmonary fibrosis	urine paraquat
Organic solvents	Benzene	marrow suppression acute leukaemia	blood count, blood benzene, urinary phenol
	Toluene	narcosis ?chronic neurological damage	blood toluene
	Carbon tetrachloride	arrhythmias liver and renal failure	–
	Trichloroethylene	skin flush with alcohol	breath trichloro-ethylene
		arrhythmias	urine trichloro-ethanol
	Carbon disulphide	psychological changes peripheral neuropathy ischaemic heart disease	urine 2-thio-thiazolidine
	Methyl butyl ketone, n-hexane	peripheral neuropathy	urine 2,5 hexanedione

those few who do rarely know how to go about it.

Why should one wish to visit the workplace? There are three reasons related to investigation of illness:

- to seek a cause of the patient's illness
- to see if the cause can be eliminated
- to see whether others are affected

There are also serious problems that make it difficult for the doctor to do this:

- ethical problems
- unfamiliarity with the approach to management
- industrial relations problems
- lack of time
- ignorance of how to go about it

Usually a combination of these factors results in no visit being made, and an opportunity to prevent disease in others is lost.

When should the workplace be visited?

The occupational physician should see regular workplace visits as much a part of the job as clinical examinations, with a view to spotting hazards and reducing risks before injury occurs. But what about the doctor who happens to see a patient with a suspected occupational disease? When should the extra, time-consuming step to visit the workplace be taken?

The short answer is whenever possible (but the visit does not have to be made by the doctor who is looking after the patient – see below, page 56). Usually the reason for the visit is not to investigate the cause – this is only necessary when the cause is suspected but not known – but to help in rehabilitation of the patient and to prevent disease in others. Of course, there are many circumstances when a visit is neither practicable nor necessary – for example in the case of diagnosis of a well-known disease such as coalworkers' pneumoconiosis when the industry concerned is already aware of and addressing the problem, or in the case of an occupational cancer due to work many years previously. However, in many cases of obvious occupational disease, such as dermatitis or back injury, failure to make any contact with the workplace means that the chance to prevent the same problems in others is missed. Indeed, in such circumstances, the medical management of the problem is of little effect if the underlying cause is not corrected.

How to make contact with the workplace

Case history 3.5

In a lecture to 25 general practitioners, one of the authors discussed a local health problem, allergies in the fish processing industry. During the discussion period, a member of the audience said that it was commonplace to see patients in his surgery with rhinitis and wheeze attributed to work in one of the prawn processing factories. They rarely responded satisfactorily to treatment and usually ended up leaving their job. He appreciated the problem, but did not know how to do anything about it.

What would have been the appropriate action? This was the question that the lecturer put back to the class.

Two hands went up. The first doctor suggested a visit to the factory, but when asked how he would approach it, he was unsure. The other doctor suggested contacting the local doctor of the Health and Safety Executive's Employment Medical Advisory Service (EMAS). When the class was asked who had heard of EMAS, three hands went up.

This event was one of the factors in deciding to write this book. In all other areas of medicine, if a doctor does not know how to handle a situation, the way out is clear – seek the advice of a colleague more expert in the area. But when it comes to occupational problems, this simple lesson is forgotten. Occupational medicine, because of its traditional separation from the mainstream of the National Health Service in Britain, is not looked upon as an accessible resource. And yet since the mid-1970s, there has been a nationwide group of doctors specifically available for advice on such matters.

Sources of advice

The most important source in Britain is the Employment Medical Advisory Service (EMAS), described more fully in Chapter 5. A phone call to the local branch of the Health and Safety Executive, asking for the Employment Medical Advisor, is all that is necessary. In doing this, it is of course important to obtain the patient's agreement to this confidential medical referral. The EMAS doctor may wish to see the patient and will take all necessary subsequent steps, including visiting the workplace, examining other workers at risk and, if necessary, arranging a visit by the Factory Inspector.

There are alternative approaches that a doctor might wish to take. If the workplace already has its own occupational health service, the doctor should approach the physician in charge, who could then make the investigation. That doctor in turn should advise his employer to make a report to EMAS if the condition is a reportable one (see Chapter 4 and Appendix 1). Or the doctor might wish to consult a university department of occupational medicine, an NHS consultant in occupational medicine, or an independent consultant. Finally, the doctor may wish to visit the workplace him- or herself.

Problems in arranging a workplace visit

Ethics (see also Chapter 10)

The relationship between a doctor and patient is confidential, and it is not acceptable to disclose information obtained from that relationship to a third party without the patient's permission. There may be particular dangers, perceived or real, to disclosure of clinical information to an agent of the employer, in that the worker may fear loss of job or some other form of discrimination. Even disclosure to another doctor, as to one in EMAS, may allow identification of individuals and their complaints by management. However, on the other side is the doctor's duty to do everything reasonably practicable for the health of the patient and to prevent disease in others.

The solution to this conundrum lies in clear explanation of the care to be taken to preserve confidentiality and to protect the patient from possible discriminatory action prior to seeking permission for referral or agreement to make a visit. Two points can be made here – in almost all cases, if the patient desires confidentiality it can be maintained (and if it cannot, the patient will withhold agreement) and, in general, managers are anxious not to cause injury to their employees and will be extremely cooperative in acting to prevent further trouble. Furthermore, if they are not, their legal obligations under the Health and Safety at Work, etc. Act (see Chapter 5) can be pointed out to them.

Ethical problems are avoided by clear explanation to the patient of the doctor's desire to help by preventing further harm and of the confidential nature of communications between doctors. With the patient's permission, it is then possible to refer the problem to a specialist who will discuss with the patient further approaches to the workplace and to management. Only if the patient's permission is given, can management be informed of the clinical problem, and then only in general terms. This should not of course hinder the doctor in the workplace from giving explicit advice to managers on preventive measures to protect workers.

The approach to management

If the company employs a doctor, the best approach is directly to him or her. If not, it is usual to speak to the most senior person on the site, normally the factory manager. The reasons for requesting a visit should be clearly explained, namely an anxiety that something in the workplace may be causing illness among the workers, and an eagerness to help in preventing future problems. It is both sensible and good medicine to stress this positive objective, since management will have fears about an approach from outside – fears of litigation and trade union disputes, and fears of unrealistic demands on the budget in order to put things right.

Workers' representatives

In general, and in contrast to their popular image, trade unionists are helpful and cooperative when it comes to dealing with possible health hazards in the workplace. There is, however, a risk that individuals may take the opportunity of fomenting industrial unrest if they suspect such a problem but have not been fully informed. For this reason, as also for ethical reasons, it is advisable that the workforce's representatives should be made aware of the visit and taken into management's confidence about the reasons, the arrangements, and the means of reporting the outcome. In most larger workplaces, the workers will have appointed safety representatives who sit on the factory safety committee with managers. This is often a useful forum for discussion of possible hazards to health, though again care has to be taken to preserve the confidentiality of individuals. Lay people are often ignorant of the ethical responsibilities of doctors, and may ask inappropriate questions.

The visit

Arrangements

The initial approach should be followed by a meeting with appropriate managers to discuss the purpose of the visit and the anticipated outcome. The advisability of discussion with unions or workers' representatives should be brought up and normally a joint meeting arranged. This gives an opportunity to allay fears and suspicions and to make clear that the purpose of a medical visit is to help prevent possible health problems.

The initial meeting with management should also be used to learn about the factory or workplace – in the case of the manufacturing industry, the raw materials, the processes, the products and by-products, waste and pollutants and the workforce. A brief check-list is given in Table 3.6.

Table 3.6   The workplace visit – important information

What raw materials are used?
How are they processed?
What are the products?
What byproducts are there?
How are waste and pollutants removed?
How big is the workforce?
What is the shift pattern?
Which workers work in the different areas/processes?
Who comes into contact with hazards?
Who does the repair/maintenance?
What safety precautions are taken?
How are these affected by repair/maintenance?
Are contract workers employed?
How do their working conditions differ from those ofthe regular workers?

In service industries, this matter is simplified in that the complex questions about processes are unnecessary and the emphasis is on environmental hazards, usually related to the building, and on methods of work organization.

In many industries, the process is complex and difficult for a non-specialist to understand. All such organizations have a flow diagram, often in the control room, which allows an outsider to obtain an overview of what goes on.

Looking around

This, the vital part of the visit, is best done in a structured way. It varies in complexity, from a short look at the particular process thought to be responsible for trouble to a detailed examination of a whole industry. The former is more usual for the clinical doctor, the latter for the epidemiologist and occupational physician. The visit should of course be made in the company of someone who understands the workplace and the processes. The factory general manager usually has most overall knowledge, though the production manager will have often more detailed knowledge of processes. The safety manager or safety officer has a particular responsibility for health and safety matters and the personnel manager (to whom the safety officer commonly reports) is most knowledgeable about the workforce, sickness absence and welfare matters. In service industries, personnel and safety managers and, often, engineers and building officers are useful contacts.

The simplest method of making a visit, having learnt about the process, is to follow it through from the entry of raw materials to the dispatch of the final product. It is important to watch what people actually do and to ask what happens when the process breaks down or shuts down. Particular attention should be paid to the handling of materials and chemicals and to possible exposure to airborne hazards. Of course, the doctor making a visit will be influenced by the condition of the patient or patients that provoked the visit, and here special attention would be paid to the particular job in question. If the likely cause is found, an assessment should be made of whether other workers are at risk (and not necessarily only on the shift during which the visit took place).

Watching the patient, or a colleague of the patient, do the job is an extension of the occupational history (Fig. 3.6). Workers vary in the care they take, just as organizations vary in their protective measures. In the investigation of dermatitis, for example, a very fastidious worker may be found to be at greater risk because of repeated washing of the hands, while some less hygienic people may become sensitized as a consequence of contaminating their cigarettes with allergenic chemicals. In some instances, quite unexpected procedures come to light on a workplace visit.

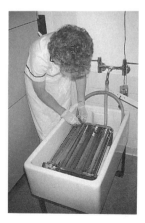

Fig. 3.6 Washing a unit from the X-ray processor. Normally this is enclosed but has to be removed on a regular basis for cleaning, allowing exposure to chemical vapours

Case history 3.6

A doctor was asked to advise an organization about safety in its animal laboratories. A careful examination of the workplace showed a number of areas in which there was a risk of skin and lung sensitization to people working on rodents. Appropriate recommendations were made. Some months later, the same doctor was asked to investigate an outbreak of skin disease in a biochemical laboratory in the same organization. While the technicians were showing him the way they did their work, one of their colleagues brought a live rat into the laboratory and proceeded to anaesthetize it on the bench. At the time, 5 other people were working in the small laboratory; all were therefore at risk of developing occupational asthma, even though only one actually worked with rats.

The doctor dealt with the dermatitis problem and went back, a chastened man, to rewrite the animal house codes of practice. He had assumed that all work with rodents took place in the designated part of the animal laboratory and had forgotten that human beings often put convenience before safety!

The investigation of workplaces often brings to light the use of substances, often chemicals, which are not known to the doctor. Frequently their identity is concealed by trade names or by their presence in complex mixtures. However, all chemicals used in industry should be subject to a data sheet, provided by the maker or supplier, which gives appropriate physical, chemical and toxicological data, together with advice on any precautions to be taken and action when accidental exposure occurs. Furthermore, in Britain, regulations on the Control of Substances Hazardous to Health (COSHH, see Chapter 5) require employers to have made an assessment of risk from the use of any hazardous substances, and to have made a written record of this assessment. These documents should be available for inspection. If further information on such substances is required, a list of readily accessible sources is given in Appendix 3.

The outcome of the visit

The visit should lead to three outcomes:

- confirmation of the hazard and assessment of risk
- action to reduce risk
- identification of others affected or at risk.

Once a hazard has been identified, it may be necessary to study it in more detail prior to planning preventive measures. This requires the use of the techniques of occupational hygiene and ergonomics.

Occupational hygiene is a discipline which applies scientific methods to investigation and measurement of hazards in the workplace and to control of risks from those hazards.

Ergonomics is a discipline devoted to the study of people in relation to their work and workplace.

These disciplines are discussed further in Chapter 5. All occupational physicians learn something of them – essentially an occupational hygienist is concerned with chemical, noise and radiation hazards and with their measurement and control, while an ergonomist is concerned with workplace, machinery and system design so as to ensure that a person's work is as well suited to his or her capabilities as possible. An occupational hygienist might be consulted, for example, for advice on control of airborne hazards from laboratory animals, an ergonomist for assistance in design of manual work so as to reduce risk of backache.

The measures taken to reduce risk and to manage individuals with occupational disease are discussed in Chapter 4. The workplace visit should allow these measures to be planned so that, ideally, the patient can return to the job and others will not be affected. In some cases, the visit may point to the need for a more extensive study of the workforce – this requires the epidemiological approach.

Epidemiological investigation

Epidemiology involves the study of groups of people in order to determine patterns of health and ill-health within these groups. Analysis of the data derived from such studies may show relationships between disease (or health) and the environment, and lead to action to modify these relationships so as to improve health. This important outcome is often not considered by many doctors, whose curiosity is satisfied when a probably causative relationship is demonstrated. As can be seen from the best-known example of epidemiology – the demonstration of a relationship between smoking and lung cancer – this is often because the action required to prevent disease is usually largely out of the hands of doctors and depends more on politicians and other policy makers.

The epidemiological process is in fact analogous to the clinical, as shown in Fig. 3.7. The clinician studies a patient, makes an examination, the synthesis of which leads to a diagnosis. In turn this should lead to decisions about treatment and prognosis, each of which may modify the other. The epidemiologist studies groups of people, gathers data and makes analyses that lead to descriptions of health/disease profiles in the group. This information may then lead to predictions of likely outcome of certain environmental changes and to interventions to make these outcomes more favourable. The clinician uses deductive logic in the diagnostic process, arguing from general medical knowledge to the particular circumstances of the patient, while the epidemiologist uses inductive logic, arguing from the particular findings in the group studied in order to make more general predictions.

In occupational medicine, there are several situations where an epidemio-

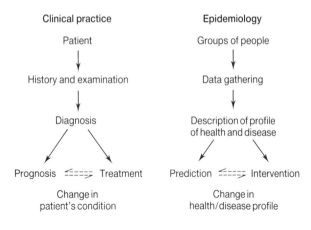

Fig. 3.7   The epidemiological investigation

logical study should be considered:

- investigation of a suspected health hazard in a well-established industry
- determination of quantitative relationships between hazard and risk of disease or injury
- measurement of the functional effects of occupational disease
- assessing the effectiveness of preventive measures.

The doctor involved in occupational medicine must be prepared to think broadly about the investigation of problems. Much may be learned from the investigation of individual patients, the clinical approach. Often epidemiology is necessary to answer questions raised by the clinician, though for epidemiology to be of immediate value a workforce must have been exposed to an adverse environment for long enough for measurable effects to have occurred. If this is not the case, it may be necessary to apply toxicological methods to the investigation of suspect substances. Often, a combination may be required and in occupational epidemiology it is always important that some assessment or measurement of the workplace or exposure is included in addition to measurement of effects on people. This is so for two reasons: first the demonstration of an exposure-response relationship is important evidence of causation and, second, since many hazards cannot be eliminated, quantitative information can be used in setting standards to reduce the risk to a level acceptable to those concerned.

Case history 3.7

A worker in a factory making PVC had a chest radiograph which was reported as showing fine diffuse nodularity. At the time there was much anxiety in the industry after the discovery of the association of hepatic angiosarcoma with exposure to vinyl chloride monomer in the retorts prior to polymerization, and it was feared that there might also be harmful effects on the lung. The factory doctor therefore arranged for the entire workforce to be X-rayed and invited a specialist to report on the films. A proportion were said to show minor abnormalities. Anxiety was increased further, so a second expert was asked to read the films. This doctor found fewer abnormalities, and showed little agreement with the first reader, of whose results he was unaware.

The factory doctor now had a problem! What did he tell the workforce, and what did he do about the individuals whose films were reported abnormal by one or other reader? What would you have done?

In fact, the factory doctor decided to ask a third doctor, an 'even bigger expert', to read the films. Fortunately, this doctor asked the vital question – 'What do you want to know?' The factory doctor was encouraged to formulate a question in terms that could be answered epidemiologically. The first response was 'Does exposure to PVC cause pneumoconiosis?' This question could be answered experimentally, by studies for example on rats, but not convincingly epidemiologically. It would, however, be possible to demonstrate whether or not there was a relationship between exposures in the workplace to PVC dust and presence of radiographic change. If such a relationship existed, then it might be possible to make recommendations on levels of dust that would reduce the risk. It would also be possible to compare other measures of ill-health, such as lung function, in people with and without such radiographic change and thus comment on the physiological consequences of the abnormalities.

A cross-sectional chest X-ray survey was carried out of the current workforce and of a sample of those who had left the factory over the previous decade. Measurements of current exposures to dust were made by personal dust samplers, and estimates of the workers' total dust exposures were calculated from these, together with detailed individual job histories. Chest radiographs were read, according to a standardized format, by several readers independently, and the results used to describe relationships between dust exposure and prevalence of radiographic change (Fig. 3.8). The company was then able to discuss the findings with the workforce and with government authorities, and agree on appropriate dust standards to protect people from possible harm.

This case history illustrates the essentially practical nature of occupational epidemiology, and also points out the essential steps in such a study. These include:

- definition of the question in terms that can be addressed epidemiologically
- definition of the population to be studied
- choosing an appropriate study design
- standardizing the methods of measurement
- obtaining a good participation rate.

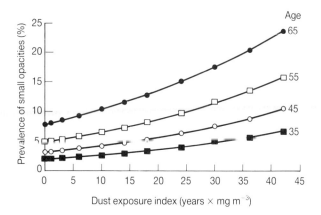

Fig. 3.8 Exposure-response relationship derived from cross-sectional study of PVC workers showing estimated increases in risk of early x-ray changes in relation to increasing current exposure to PVC dust

Defining the question

Research starts with a hypothesis to be tested, an idea or a question to which the answer is not known. Such questions arise commonly in clinical practice, if the doctor is of an inquisitive turn of mind. Often the answer may be found by searching the medical literature, but sometimes this is unsuccessful – the answer is not known. In occupational medicine, such problems fall into two groups: those in which people have been exposed to an agent for a sufficient period for measurable effects to have appeared and those in which they have not (yet). In the latter case, toxicological research is necessary, but in the former epidemiological techniques are appropriate.

The question is usually a clinical one, such as 'What has caused these patients' nasal cancers?' or 'Why have I seen so many cases of cerebellar ataxia among painters?' These questions need to be changed into a format that allows an epidemiological approach, and this requires a hypothesis. In the case of the nasal cancer, for example, an ear, nose and throat surgeon was impressed by having seen several such cases among workers in the furniture trade, leading to the hypothesis that exposure to dust in that trade was responsible for the tumour. She was then able to plan studies of groups of such workers to test this hypothesis and ultimately to show clear evidence of a relationship between such work and nasal cancer. The question about cerebellar ataxia in painters might be reframed as a hypothesis that exposure to paint solvents causes the disease. This then could be tested by appropriate studies either of people with (cases) and without (controls) cerebellar ataxia or of populations of painters or solvent-exposed workers.

Since epidemiology is rarely able to establish causation firmly, questions are normally framed in terms of relationships and probabilities and the answers stated in terms of statistical likelihood. Thus the question will usually be of the form 'Is there a relationship between disease and hypothetical cause and, if so, what is the likelihood of that relationship having occurred by chance?', or 'How frequently have people with a certain disease been exposed to a particular agent, relative to controls?'

Defining the population

All epidemiological studies are studies of groups of people, of populations. Many badly designed studies are inconclusive because of a failure to define the population at risk; it is clearly not possible to know the prevalence of a condition without knowing how many people are at risk for it.

The total population at risk may be called the *target population*. In the case of painters with cerebellar disease, this might be all painters in Britain. In practical terms, this would not be a group that could be studied, so a subgroup, such as all painters employed by a representative group of companies or working in a particular area may be chosen as the *study population*. It is important to realize that any conclusions derived from the study ultimately refer only to those people studied, and can only be generalized after taking account of any biases that may have arisen in this selection process.

In choosing the population, it is necessary to bear in mind the necessity of obtaining a good participation rate. Ideally, all those chosen as the study population should be seen, and it is generally held that a response of below 90 per cent of this considerably weakens any conclusions drawn. This is because it becomes less and less easy to estimate bias arising from non-participation – is it because the ill did not attend or because the well could not be bothered? The most challenging and time-consuming aspect of epidemiology is that concerned with ensuring a complete response.

Designing the study

Few things are more disappointing than to have done a great deal of work only to find out that it is valueless. This, regrettably, is the fate of many who rush into an epidemiological study without adequate thought and statistical advice. The study must clearly address the question or questions being asked, and must be planned in such a way as to have a reasonable chance of getting a positive answer or a meaningful negative one. This latter concept is known as the *statistical power* of the study. The simplest type of study, conceptually, might set out to determine the *prevalence* of a certain condition in the defined population, that is the number of people with a pre-defined condition expressed as a proportion of the numbers in the population. This is analogous to a survey of voting intentions and similarly can only be taken to be true at the time of the study. Whether the prevalence of a particular disease or finding is abnormal requires reference to a control population or to a variable, usually exposure to a toxic substance, within the study population. Thus it may be possible to show that the prevalence of skin disease is greater in hairdressers than in shop assistants, leading to further hypotheses about possible causes of this problem in hairdressers. In turn, this may be addressed by investigating the relationship within a group of hairdressers between prevalence of skin disease and exposure to agents thought to be responsible. Note that such studies are never quite as simple as they seem at first sight – are shop assistants an appropriate control population? How is skin disease defined for the purpose of the study? How may exposure to skin-damaging agents be quantified? Are there any confounding factors, such as age, use of make-up or exposure to sunlight or ultra-violet light, that might influence the results and should therefore be taken into account in the design?

A *prevalence (or cross-sectional) study* therefore examines a population in a cross-sectional manner at a given time or over a short defined period. It is usually desirable to choose a population defined retrospectively, say all workers employed in the industry between certain dates, and this is especially necessary when studying conditions that develop only after a period of exposure. This method of selection allows one to avoid the trap of missing workers who have left the industry *because* they developed the condition in question, thus producing a spuriously low prevalence in the current population. Such cross-sectional studies should therefore include at least a sample of retired workers from the defined population. Prevalence studies are useful for defining relationships between disease and cause, where the disease or abnormality being sought is a relatively common one. If the results of such a study are to be of real value not only in contributing to understanding of cause but also in planning preventive measures, they require to incorporate measurements of hypothetical causative factors as well as response variables. For example, in the PVC case study above, exposures of workers to PVC dust were measured and this allowed the derivation of an index of exposure for each subject in the study. This was calculated from the occupational histories recorded, multiplying the concentration of dust in each job (mg/m³) by the number of years spent in each job, and adding up these increments of dust exposure for all the jobs each individual worker had done in the factory. This gave an index in mg.years/m³ for each worker, and a wide range of such exposures in the workforce, from almost nil in secretaries up to very high in some long-serving process workers. This allowed the plotting of a relationship between exposure and risk of having X-ray changes (Fig. 3.8) Such an *exposure-response relationship* is strong evidence of causality.

Where the condition is relatively rare, or where one wishes to determine the effect of a particular condition on health, a *case-control (or retrospective) study* is often more appropriate. Here, cases are defined as individuals with the disease or abnormality in question while controls are people from the same population but who do not have the disease. Both groups are then investigated in identical ways, preferably by someone who is unaware of whether the individual is a case or a control. Differences between the two groups may then be expressed in terms of the *relative risk* of one group having a particular exposure or functional abnormality compared to the other. Note the difference between controls in case-control studies and those in prevalence studies – in the former they are individuals without the condition being investigated, while in the latter they are a group without the hypothetically causative exposure.

Case history 3.8

A hospital registrar had read the suggestion that proliferative glomerulonephritis might be associated with exposure to solvents. A review of the literature showed that this hypothesis, though plausible (excretion through the kidneys could damage the nephron), was still in dispute. He had access, through the records of renal biopsy, to a reasonable number of patients with this clearly defined condition, and sought advice on an appropriate study.

If he came to you, what would you suggest? A cross-sectional study of people exposed to solvents or a case-control study?

The problem was discussed. A cross-sectional study would require identification of an appropriate population of people exposed to solvents, and a survey to determine whether or not they had evidence of renal disease, perhaps by examination of their urine. It would require either estimates of exposure to solvents or identification of an otherwise comparable non-exposed population. Clearly, this would be a time-consuming and expensive study. Moreover, calculations based on the likely prevalence of renal disease in the population suggested that, unless solvent exposure was an important cause of the disease, a very large study would be required to find an effect.

In contrast, a case-control study seemed straightforward. Cases could be defined histologically and controls could be drawn from the same population – patients referred to the hospital at the same time as cases, but who did not have glomerulonephritis. Precautions were taken to match cases and controls for two important factors that could influence the development of glomerulonephritis, age and gender, and a questionnaire on exposure to solvents and occupations was administered to cases and controls by a clerk who was unaware of the diagnosis. The results showed that the group with glomerulonephritis had a risk of having worked with or been exposed to solvents considerably greater than that of the controls, and that this difference was unlikely to be due to chance.

A major problem in case-control studies is the choice of controls. In order to avoid bias, they should be drawn from the same original population and, were it not for the factor under investigation, should have had an equal chance of getting the disease. The cases have the disease, the controls not and the study seeks to determine risk factors associated with having the disease. Any factor which independently influences the chances of having the disease and the risk factor being investigated is called a *confounder*, and cases and controls should be matched for this. In the example above, age and gender were regarded as counfounders. Other matching is best avoided, as overmatching can result in possible risk factors being eliminated – for example, matching on area of residence will eliminate the possibility of finding a geographical factor. In hospital-based studies, other patients attending the clinic or clinics may be suitable controls, but care should be taken to allow for differing referral patterns to different doctors. Other studies may use relatives, neighbours or random samples from the same general practice or electoral roll as controls. In planning case-control studies, as in all epidemiology, the involvement of a statistician is crucial.

The other common use of a case-control study is to investigate the functional effects of a disease. The same problems of control selection obtain, but the comparison is here made in terms of measured function, be it physical abnormality, liver or lung function, or whatever.

A third type of study is the *longitudinal (or cohort) study*. This measures the *incidence or attack rate* of a disease or abnormality over a defined period of time. In one form, it may measure mortality.

Case history 3.9

During a period of crisis in the world oil market, the United States Government decided to investigate the possibility of exploiting its reserves of oil shale in the Rocky Mountains. Since shale oil had been known to be carcinogenic from the days of the late Industrial Revolution, it was considered advisable to take precautions to protect the workers, both miners and process workers. But what risks would these people run, and from what substances?

How might risks be assessed in a new, or fairly new industry? What options can you think of?

> The US risk assessment team considered animal experiments and cytotoxicity tests of substances likely to be produced in the industry. They also considered analogy with other similar industries. But what they really needed to know was the effects of previous oil shale industries on the health of their workforce. Fortunately, it was possible to identify a cohort of several thousand men who had been working in the Scottish oil shale industry in 1950, prior to its final closure in 1962. It proved possible to identify which of these men were alive and which dead and, in the case of the latter, to identify the cause of death. After appropriate corrections for age, it was then possible to relate the risk of mortality from different conditions in these workers to the risk of members of the general population of Scotland. The results of such analyses, expressed as age-standardized mortality ratios and their 95 per cent confidence intervals, showed that the Scottish workers had an increased risk of premature death from skin cancer but from no other disease. In particular, lung cancer was shown not to have occurred more frequently than expected.

The results of this study were useful in that they did not reveal any risks of major diseases and the power of the study made it unlikely that a real risk was missed. Similar mortality studies have been coupled with measurements or estimates of exposure, for example to asbestos, in order to predict excess risk of death associated with different levels of exposure to harmful substances. Clearly such studies are of considerable value in planning preventive strategies. They do, however, have several disadvantages:

- they are expensive and time-consuming
- they require a population to have been exposed for many years
- they rarely are able to obtain accurate information on exposure.

Two other applications of longitudinal studies are to investigate the incidence of disease and to measure changes in function over time. Both require the same criteria for identification of population together with choice of an appropriate control, be it a non-exposed population or measurement of a possible causative variable within the study population.

Case history 3.10

> Several workers in a factory producing citric acid developed asthma, and this was shown to be due to allergy to Aspergillus niger, a fungus used in the process. A cross-sectional survey was carried out and identified work-related asthma in 5 per cent of the workforce, of whom half had skin prick test evidence of allergy to *A. niger*. Extensive precautions were taken thereafter to reduce the exposure of workers to antigen, and annual surveillance of the workforce by questionnaire

and skin prick testing was carried out. Over the next 5 years it was shown that no new cases of asthma had occurred in the original cohort, nor had any new positive skin tests been found.

This example illustrates a simple use of a longitudinal survey in order to ensure that preventive measures are effective. If coupled to appropriate measurements of exposure, the results may be used to modify any exposure standards previously set. If the study design includes in addition measurements of function (in this example, lung function might have been appropriate), it may be possible to investigate the relative contributions to functional deterioration of age, smoking and exposure to antigen.

Standardizing methods of measurement

In epidemiology, as in clinical and laboratory medicine, the measurements made should be capable of producing the same result when repeated by the same or by another observer; in other words, intra-and inter-observer error must be small. Thus, when making observations on large numbers of people in an epidemiological population, the tests to be used should be carefully standardized in order to minimize variability. The same applies to methods used in the measurement of the workplace environment. Furthermore, the methods should have been, or should be able to be, validated, so that the results derived should show some relationship to other standard measurement. Table 3.7 shows some of the methods and terms used in such validation.

Table 3.7   Validation of a test

	Standard method Positive	Negative	Study method Totals
Study method positive negative	true positives (a) false negatives (c)	false positives (b) true negatives (d)	positives (a + b) negatives (c + d)
true totals	positives (a + c)	negatives (b + d)	

sensitivity of study method $= \dfrac{a}{a + c}$

specificity of study method $= \dfrac{d}{b + d}$

systematic error (ratio of study method positives to true positives)

$$= \frac{a + b}{a + c}$$

positive predictive value (proportion of study method positives that are truly positive)

$$= \frac{a}{a + b}$$

For many tests, the 'true' value is not directly measurable and the test may have to be validated indirectly. For example (a well-known one), the rather arbitrary classification of X-ray changes of pneumoconiosis based on comparison of films of workers with standard films selected by a panel of experts has been validated more effectively by relating the results of epidemiological surveys to indices of dust exposure in the populations than by direct comparison of films with pathological changes in the lungs of individuals after death. The logic of this is illustrated below.

Case history 3.11

It had long been known that workers in certain dusty trades were at risk of developing pneumoconiosis, a condition characterized by small, and sometimes large, opacities on the chest radiograph. Various methods of classifying such shadows had been developed in different countries so that epidemiological studies of prevalence, incidence, progression and influence of preventive measures could be made. For results to be generalisable, standardized methods were necessary for use in different industries worldwide.

After several international discussions, it was decided that standard films would be selected that illustrated different stages and types of pneumoconiosis, each being selected as an individual point on a continuum of change, from normal to extremely abnormal. Consensus was reached on the choice of films, which were then used in many international studies of dust-exposed workers. The films were validated by their use in studies of, for example, coalminers and asbestos workers, wherein it was shown that the higher exposure a worker had suffered, the greater the risk of the film showing more advanced changes. Thus it can now be stated that profusion of radiological change is an indirect measure of dust exposure.

These studies have also shown that the standard films are far from perfect, and have to be used with great caution as a *diagnostic*, as opposed to an epidemiological, tool. Inter-and intra-reader variability is often considerable, and small opacities are related to factors, age and smoking habits for example, other than dust exposure. Further discussions are regularly convened to improve these methods of categorizing X-ray changes.

The most frequent epidemiological tool in occupational medicine is the questionnaire. The design of a questionnaire is complex, and as far as possible investigators are encouraged to use one that has already been used and shown to produce reproducible answers and to be valid. If a new one needs to be designed, a few points should be borne in mind.

- The questions should be: short
  comprehensible by the group to be studied
  unambiguous
- The questions should not: suggest an answer
  combine two or more questions in one

- The questionnaire: should have a logical order
                        should include clear routing instructions

Examples of bad questions are:

Do you ever suffer from an itch or redness of the skin?

These two questions should be asked separately, as subsequent questions could refer to either or both symptoms.

Have you ever suffered from hypertension?

Many people will not understand terms that are familiar to doctors – high blood pressure is better here.

Is your cough worse when you are at work?

This suggests a cause of the cough and introduces a bias into the study. It is better to ask:

Does your cough vary during the week?

If yes:

On which day or days is it worse? and
On which day or days is it better?

This can be achieved simply by providing a box for each day of the week and asking the subject to tick the boxes for the days on which the symptom is most troublesome.

In designing a questionnaire, after the questions have been decided upon (and they should generally be the smallest number consistent with achieving the aims of the study), the logic of the routing instructions should be checked. The rule is to have the subject answer only relevant questions, so if a 'no' is recorded to presence of a symptom, supplementary questions are avoided and the subject or questionner is directed to the next relevant one. The usual method of checking is to administer the draft questionnaire to a friend or relative. Mistakes will be found and after these have been corrected, a pilot study should be made on a group of people from similar social background to the intended study population, to pick up ambiguities and incomprehensible terms.

Administration of a questionnaire may be by a trained clerk (who should know not to explain, elaborate or prompt) or by the subjects themselves. Many practical difficulties attend such surveys, chief of which is obtaining an adequate response rate.

Obtaining a good participation rate

No matter how good the methods and design, an epidemiological study is easily rendered valueless by a poor rate of participation by the subjects, just as a poll of voting intentions is rendered uncertain by a high proportion of 'don't knows' or 'mind-your-own-businesses'. The key to success is hard work – in designing a study that will be acceptable to the subjects, in publicizing the study and obtaining agreement and support from key people (such as union representatives) in the study population, and in tracing individuals and politely inviting their participation. In occupational epidemiology, where there is often a readily definable workplace population, the most important steps are those taken in explaining the purpose of the survey to the subjects beforehand and in telling them how and when the results will be communicated to them. Any hint of secrecy, and the study is doomed to failure. Problems arise with tracing and follow-up of retired workers, and here the help of older workers and union or personnel/pension records is invaluable.

Screening for disease

The surveillance of workers for the presence of disease is considered further in Chapter 5. At this point, it is worth noting a few principles, relating to the value of and justification for screening. The following questions should be asked before embarking on a screening programme:

- Is the condition important for individuals or the community?
- Is there effective treatment for/management of the condition?
- Is the condition's natural history, especially its evolution from latent to overt, understood?
- Is there a recognisable latent or early stage?
- Is there a valid and reproducible screening test?
- Are facilities available for management of the positive findings, both true or false?
- Is there an agreed management policy?
- Does this management favourably influence the course of the disease?
- Is the cost of case-finding and management acceptable in relation to the overall costs of health care?
- Do the potential benefits to true positives outweigh the potential disadvantages for the false positives?

It is clear that any thoughtful person would pause before introducing general health screening in a workforce if such questions were considered. The chief disadvantage of 'health checks', apart from their grossly inefficient use of resources, is the harm done to individuals when insignificant findings lead to a series of unnecessary and sometimes dangerous investigations. When screening a healthy workforce, such false positives are likely greatly to outnumber true positives for whom useful intervention is possible.

Determining the cause of disease

As outlined at the start of this chapter, the cause of disease in an individual may be determined clinically by, for example, patch testing or bronchial challenge. In epidemiology, studies point to relationships between ill health and possibly causative or contributory environmental factors. It is however ultimately possible to accumulate sufficient evidence to make a causal relationship extremely likely. The late Sir Austen Bradford Hill proposed widely accepted criteria by which the evidence should be judged:

1. How *strong* is the association, or how unlikely
    is it to have occurred by chance?
2. How *consistent* are all the studies that have
    investigated the association?
3. Is the condition apparently *specific* to a group
    exposed to a particular agent?
4. Is there a *temporal relationship* between proposed
    cause and the effect?
5. Is there an *exposure-response relationship* between
    cause and effect?
6. Is the relationship *biologically plausible?*
7. Is the evidence *coherent*, in that it does not conflict
    with known facts about the condition's natural history?
8. Is the evidence supported by *experimental evidence*
    in laboratories?
9. Does the evidence accord, by *analogy*, with that
    derived from other fields?

Two examples serve to illustrate the value of these tests; hepatic angiosarcoma in vinyl chloride workers and lung cancer in silica-exposed workers. In the case of the former, the first five criteria are fully satisfied, the sixth was originally uncertain (was a simple anaesthetic agent likely to cause liver cancer?) but was settled with inhalation studies in rats (criterion 8), and criteria 7 and 9 are unimportant in the face of all the other evidence. In the case of silica and lung cancer, the evidence of association is becoming stronger and more consistent, although the disease is certainly not specific to silica workers; increasing evidence is being produced in support of criteria 4 to 7, and there is now some, weak, experimental evidence of causation. It may be concluded that vinyl chloride causes angiosarcoma, but that the case against silica remains unproven – if it has a role in causing lung cancer, it must be a relatively weak one in epidemiological terms.

4

The management of occupational disease

Summary

This chapter discusses the management of patients with occupational disease. In the practice of occupational medicine there is rarely a place for prescription of drugs or other therapeutic intervention, save in the case of certain workplace emergencies. The role of the doctor in these, and in ensuring the provision of appropriate first aid services, as well as liaison with local hospitals and other doctors is discussed.

Besides the immediate management of occupational disease, doctors have wider responsibilities in preventing recurrence in the affected individual and occurrence of similar episodes in other employees. Thus the diagnosis of occupational disease should often lead to modification of the job and/or the workplace. While the doctor in industry is well placed to recommend this, doctors in hospital or in general practice may often need to seek specialist help from the Employment Medical Advisory Service (the medical arm of the Health and Safety Executive) or from other occupational physicians.

Another important responsibility of the doctor diagnosing occupational disease is to ensure that legal reporting requirements are met, although in Britain the actual report of specific reportable diseases must be made by the employer. Finally doctors should be able to advise their patients on matters concerning statutory compensation and, depending on their expertise, issues of causality where a civil action is being pursued.

Introduction

Occupational disease constitutes only a small, but often underestimated, proportion of the workload of general practitioners or hospital doctors. When workers are ill, their occupation is not commonly the cause and when work is the cause of injury or disease the occupational physician's contribution to treatment in the narrow clinical sense is limited. Nevertheless, there are important specific aspects of the management of occupational disease, whether it is an emergency or not, that are sometimes neglected, perhaps through ignorance. The purpose of this chapter is to fill these gaps for the benefit of any physician who may come across occupational disease. Some points are covered in other chapters but bear reinforcing. Thus the first contribution of the medical profession should be to assist in the prevention of occupational disease (Chapter 5). Second, detection of occupational disease should be as early as possible (Chapter 3) since this will usually have advantages in the clinical outcome for the afflicted individual, as well as encouraging steps to be taken to protect other workers. Third, both the individual with occupational disease as well as his work environment need to be thoroughly assessed. Physicians should be adequately trained in these skills but at the same time must recognize their individual limitations and know where and when to seek further help. Fourth, a few aspects of treatment may be relatively specific to occupational disease. Finally, the physician also has responsibility in the statutory processes for reporting occupational disease, and in advising workers or their agents in connection with compensation.

It should therefore be clear from the foregoing and from the examples that follow that the description of the problem in occupational medicine is often more complex than in other clinical specialties where, in simple terms, the physician may merely ask: What is the diagnosis? How do I treat it? In occupational medicine, the doctor has a wider responsibility, having not only to assess the clinical problem but also to investigate the environmental factors that contributed to it, to take action to prevent further harm to the patient and to others in the same environment, and sometimes to make a formal report. The process of clinical decision-making in occupational medicine may be summarized as in Fig. 4.1.

Clinical assessment of occupational disease

The important steps in the diagnosis and investigation of occupational diseases have been dealt with in the preceding chapters. However, in many situations it is necessary not only to determine the nature and severity of a condition and its cause but it is also essential to assess the risk of its occurrence or recurrence following workplace exposure to the hazard. This assessment will help to decide the best form of management and will serve as a baseline for subsequent review of the response to its management, or in the event of later relapse. Moreover, proper assessment is important for legal purposes especially when compensation may be sought. In some cases, the clinical presentation might not initially point to an occupational cause as for example with backpain or an anxiety state, and the patient might at the time believe there to be no occupational contribution to the symptoms. Nevertheless, the physician should still assess any potential occupational exposure that might contribute, since the question of such a component to the illness with implications for its management might arise later. Detailed accounts of how to assess disease which may have similar manifestations whether or not it is work related can be found in textbooks of general medicine. A few relevant points, however, will be mentioned, since occasionally physicians in industry do not place enough emphasis on these issues.

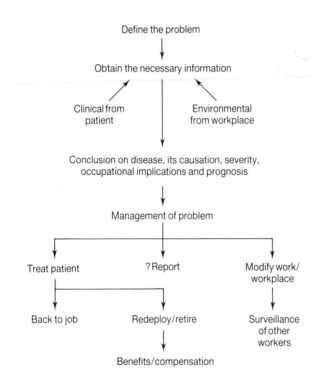

Figure 4.1   Clinical decision making in occupational medicine.

Case history 4.1.

A 28 year-old apprentice joiner had gone off sick with back pain. When seen by the physician he said that the pain had resulted from lifting a narrow wooden architrave (about 5 cm wide and 2.3 m long). On examination the doctor noted that he had some difficulty in touching his toes and on that basis concluded that he was not yet fit to return to work. He remained off work, took analgesics until he was completely pain free and then returned to exactly the same job.

The above assessment and action, though commonplace, are far from ideal. What further information should have been obtained in order to assess the severity of his illness, the prognosis and the action necessary to reduce risk of recurrence on returning to his job?

Five important matters should have been considered:

- the history of the task
- the clinical examination
- the assessment of the workplace
- statutory matters (reporting, benefits, etc.).
- rehabilitation and secondary prevention.

The history should have been assessed in detail. Thus it transpired that the wooden architrave was mixed in with a variety of other timbers which were stored at ground level. The sliding out of the desired one, with a bent and stooped back, against the resistance of the other pieces was clearly a risky task. The workplace merited detailed assessment to ensure that the wood was in future stored, properly sorted, at a higher and more accessible level.

The objective assessment was not adequate as described. Thus for example, in assessing a worker who is complaining of low back pain, one important measurement that may be important in prognosis and subsequent management is that of lumbar spinal flexion. One of the ways of determining this is by the skin marking method. Briefly, with the patient erect a line is drawn in the midline at the level of the dimples of Venus (Posterior Superior Iliac Spines), a further mark is made in the midline 10 cm above this and another 5 cm below. The patient is asked to flex as far as comfortably possible while the origin of the measuring tape is held against the top line. The more the lumbar spine can flex, the greater the skin distraction. Most normal people will easily yield to a distance beyond 20 cm between the uppermost and lowermost mark (i.e. 5 cm more than the 15 cm baseline). Additionally, clinical assessment to exclude acute lumbar intervertebral disc prolapse, including nerve stretch tests, tendon reflexes and tests of sensation should have been carried out.

The physician should have notified the manager that once at least 3 days of sickness absence had elapsed the incident was reportable as an 'Injury' under the RIDDOR (Reporting of Injuries, Diseases and Dangerous Occurrences Regulations) regulations. In more prolonged absences issues of statutory benefits (see also Chapter 7) would need to be reviewed. Finally consideration should have been given to the need to plan rehabilitation if or when appropriate (see also Chapter 8).

Case history 4.2

A 20 year-old woman started a job as an animal house technician, dealing mainly with rodents. Workplace exposure had not been properly assessed nor adequately controlled as is required by health and safety law (see Chapter 5). About 5 months later she developed symptoms of conjunctivitis, rhinitis and asthma which improved on spells away from work. Her general practitioner prescribed treatment with bronchodilators but her symptoms persisted. Eventually, after about one year in employment she had an episode of angio-oedema for which she was seen in a hospital casualty department, but no specific action in relation to her job was considered. After this episode she did not return to that work, and eventually resigned her employment.

Arguably, from a medical standpoint the problem was solved. The occupational nature of her symptoms was shown, at least circumstantially; she would no longer work in the animal house and her symptoms would be expected to resolve. However, was the management of this occupational disease really adequate? What problems can you see in the way in which the case was handled, and how might these have been resolved?

The assessment was incomplete. In all cases of asthma, questions should be asked about possible provoking causes, including occupational factors. If such factors are suspected, frequent measurements of peak flow rate, as discussed in Chapter 3, should be made.

The management of the patient was unsatisfactory. As the symptoms persisted in spite of treatment, further investigation should have taken place. Usually in such an example, referral for a second opinion is advisable; this might have been to an specialist Occupational Physician such as, in Britain, the local Employment Medical Adviser of the Health and Safety Executive (see Chapter 3).

There was no attempt to manage the overall problem. Although the patient's problem was reduced (albeit by loss of her job), the workplace problem remained, and other people in the animal house remained at risk. This important aspect of the case can only be addressed by a visit to the workplace, and it is here that the advice of a specialist is particularly important.

The patient lost her job, without financial compensation. In Britain and many other countries, there are systems for industrial injury benefits to be paid to people suffering from certain occupational diseases. The patient in this case should have been advized that her condition was one that would, in the UK, be recognized for such benefits were she to apply to the Department of Social Security. This is discussed later in the chapter.

The disease was not initially reported to the statutory authorities. Again, regulations differ in different countries, but in Britain RIDDOR put the responsibility on employers to report any of a long list of occupational diseases (see Appendix 1). The doctor who makes the diagnosis should inform the employer with the patient's consent or if this is not freely given, consult with an Employment Medical Adviser in the Health and Safety Executive directly. The regulatory authority is then in a position to take appropriate action. If this step is taken, it is often possible for the workplace risk to be reduced and for the patient to return to work.

In summary, this case contrasts what usually happens with the many issues that often need to be considered in the management of occupational disease. Both the general practitioner and the casualty officer could have obtained enough evidence to take appropriate action, to the benefit of both the patient and her workmates.

Case history 4.3

A 55 year-old woman had worked for several years in high street dry cleaning shops. In her last employment in particular she had been significantly exposed to perchlorethylene both as vapour and percutaneously. Not only did she have to clear out blocked button traps, and top up the machine with this solvent but also she was in the close vicinity of frequent leaks. She developed multiple symptoms including headaches, nausea, anxiety and Raynaud's syndrome affecting her hands. She eventually gave up the work as her symptoms worsened while exposure remained uncontrolled. Her employers did not have an occupational physician but her complaints, directly and through her general practitioner, resulted in the Health and Safety Executive investigating her workplace shortly before she left. Airborne levels of perchlorethylene were monitored and found to be in concentrations consistent with her symptoms, and the employer was obliged to take appropriate action.

Perhaps if this lady's case had been investigated earlier and appropriate steps taken to control her exposure at that time some of her symptoms could have been improved and she could have continued working for longer. However the fact that at least some investigations were carried out while she was still in employment permitted a better informed clinical management of her case as well as enabling useful data to be collected in the service of justice when she subsequently commenced litigation proceedings against her ex-employers.

Sadly, all too often employees give up their jobs spontaneously or on medical advice when there is circumstantial evidence of an association between their work and their symptoms. Investigations of occupational exposure or of specific biological markers (such as organic solvents in blood or breath, or their metabolites in urine) should be undertaken at the earliest suspicion when the symptoms may still be mild and while the worker is still in employment. Even if the circumstantial evidence is strong or the employee is considering leaving the job anyway, a good case can still be made for these investigations, which may permit identification of the specific agent, and its source, and measurement of the exposure levels responsible for the adverse health effect. They will facilitate appropriate measures to safeguard the worker's health and job and are important in stimulating action to protect other workers. This concern usually springs to mind early in the deliberations of an occupational physician, but is perhaps not so obvious to general practitioners or hospital doctors who naturally address primarily the problems of the individual in their consulting room. Finally, such investigations may provide data that will result in the courts of law being better informed should the matter eventually lead to civil or criminal action.

Assistance with these techniques should ideally be sought in the first instance from the occupational physician employed by the firm since properly trained occupational physicians are well versed in environmental and biological monitoring. However this ideal route is only available in the minority of circumstances where the firm employs such a person, and in many cases, therefore, the assistance of the Health and Safety Executive will need to be sought. Although Parliament has granted workers a right of direct access to this government organization, the concerned physician should not merely point this facility out to the patient and leave it at that. Many workers are underconfident and sometimes do not easily articulate their problem. Moreover, the Health and Safety Executive is widely held to be understaffed and may have to limit or rank its responses to cries for help. Therefore the best approach might be for the physician, after obtaining the patient's consent and armed with all the information that can be reasonably gathered (Chapter 3), to telephone the nearest local Health and Safety Executive Office and ask to speak to an Employment Medical Adviser. After these two doctors have conferred, a letter should set the seal on the conversation. The Employment Medical Adviser, who is usually a trained specialist occupational physician, would then take further steps to investigate and to manage the suspected occupational disease. These could include seeing the worker clinically and visiting the workplace alone or with a factory inspector, and in due course advising both the worker and the referring physician. Alternatively, occupational physicians employed in the National Health Service or in university academic departments will often be willing to advise a medical colleague informally although it should be stressed that this is not their official responsibility.

Besides determining the severity of overt illhealth, physicians may need to become skilled in determining the risk of illness ensuing after certain exceptional occupational exposures. These skills are important primarily for occupational physicians but also for other doctors employed in general practice or in casualty departments and who might be called upon for advice in these circumstances. In general there are two approaches, those following a 'worst case analysis' and others a 'cautious best estimate'. In the first approach one assumes that all things which could possibly go wrong will do so, and then one always implements all possible useful precautionary measures after such an event. It is generally true that, where there is doubt, it is better to be safe than sorry. However, one must not lose sight of the fact that 'crying wolf' too often is not only wasteful of time and resources and generates unnecessary anxiety but may actually put the worker at a higher risk if the intervention is inappropriate. Consider the following case history.

Case history 4.4

A hospital domestic assistant presented to the occupational health department having just injured herself with a hypodermic needle in a ward while cleaning behind a radiator. She was given Hepatitis B immunoglobulin and a course of Hepatitis B vaccine was commenced.

The above is a common scenario and one can consider the above management to have been satisfactory, but need any more have been done? A more detailed assessment should have started with inspection of the needle. A narrow bore needle as used for venepuncture to withdraw blood, or for parenteral therapy, or an intravenous cannula obviously carries a higher risk than an apparently clean wide bore needle (as used for making up drug solutions in phials). If the source was clearly identified, the Hepatitis B status of the patient on whom the needle had been used could be identified. If the ward or department was assessed one might find that it consisted of a renal dialysis unit with known Hepatitis B negative patients or a geriatric ward with low likelihood of such infection. Alternatively, if the department dealt with infectious diseases or with gastroenterology the risk would be presumed to be higher. This information should be carefully sought and recorded. Careful inspection of the needle and any syringe or other device that it may have been attached to, as well as the wound it inflicted can give a rough estimate of the size of the inoculum. Although the steps taken to prevent Hepatitis B after needlestick injury carry a very favourable risk to benefit ratio, in occupational medicine the risk to benefit ratio for other therapeutic interventions may be much less favourable or less certain and therefore diligent steps must be taken to determine the likelihood and dose of exposure before specific treatment. Examples of this include the use of the highly toxic chelating agent cobalt ethylene diamine tetracetate as a cyanide antidote or the use of zidovudine (AZT) in an attempt to prevent HIV infection after a needlestick injury, as discussed below.

First aid

A doctor working in industry has a duty not only to prevent occupational disease (as described in Chapter 5) but also to mitigate the consequences of injuries. This obligation is addressed by considering what disease, poisoning or injury could arise even after implementing preventive action. Adequate material facilities and trained personnel should be made available to deal with adverse consequences at least to a standard which complies with the relevant health and safety (first aid) regulations. These require appropriately labelled first aid boxes with a specified content to be available. In low risk workplaces the guidelines recommend one appointed person who can make arrangements for medical emergencies, but not necessarily a trained first aider, for every 50 employees. First aiders are to be identifiable and trained to a standard approved by the Health and Safety Executive, and followed up by regular 3-yearly courses so as to continue holding a valid certificate. In particular workplaces with specific hazards, first aiders should also be trained in the emergency management of such hazards. The occupational physician should be familiar with the correct assessment and management skills and then should be able to supervize the training of first aiders in this regard. Many formal training courses in first aid run by outside agencies are excellent, but are often too general and tend towards the management of trauma and nonoccupational medical emergencies rather than special occupational problems such as chemical intoxications. In contrast, the trained occupational physician should have both relevant professional knowledge and an understanding of the specific workplace hazards, and is therefore ideally placed to train the first aid team which he or she is likely to have to work with in an emergency. Moreover, the physician should liaise with the nearest casualty department to ensure that the knowledge and facilities exist to deal with any medical emergencies peculiar to that workplace such as anticholinesterase poisoning, methaemoglobinaemia, etc.

Case history 4.5

In a chemical manufacturing firm on the first occasion that recommissioned plant was in use after alteration, a process worker donned an air hood as personal protection before commencing a task that could have involved solvent exposure. He was seen to lose consciousness by a workmate who was a trained first aider. The first aider immediately pulled off the victim's air hood and carried him away from the immediate vicinity of the reactor vessel. Oxygen was administered by face mask within minutes, and by the time the occupational physician arrived, the worker was regaining consciousness; he eventually made a full and complete recovery. It was discovered that during the alterations the fitting for the air line had inadvertently and negligently been welded onto a nitrogen blanket line (used to cover certain chemical reactions with nitrogen rather than air to prevent unwanted oxidation).

It is clear that had it not been for the prompt, appropriate and effective action of the first aider the casualty would have died or suffered brain damage. The investment made in training these first aiders that, in the event of unconsciousness (of nontraumatic origin), the casualty was to be urgently but safely removed from his immediate environment, given oxygen and kept in the coma position had clearly paid dividends.

Many large and responsible firms, usually with an occupational health service, try hard to establish a good working relationship with their local hospital and general practitioners. This liaison can be lifesaving in the emergency management of occupational diseases as well as in dealing with less severe cases. Hospital doctors and general practitioners should respond positively to invitations to open days, joint meetings and such like. It is a paradox that some small firms with serious occupational hazards and no occupational health service and whose workers would therefore rely exclusively on medical skills outside the workplace in an emergency do not try hard enough to forge such links. General practitioners and hospital doctors who become aware of such workplaces, whether through 'herald' patients perhaps presenting with minor illness or in other ways should contact the workplace directly. They should ask to speak to any occupational health or safety professional if there is one or, failing this, to the manager. If this proves difficult it is better to seek the advice and help of the Health and Safety Executive early rather than wait until a serious and perhaps life-threatening incident results.

Medical treatment

Some physicians both within and outside the workplace might feel that, since the occupational physician is not responsible for the primary care of the employees, medical treatment in the strict sense is never part of this role. However, the occupational physician may have an important treatment function in emergencies, and in other occupational illness where specific training and experience can be important adjuvants to the advice of the other medical attendants. Nevertheless one should avoid the fallacy of believing that most occupational illnesses, even the acute ones, have specific remedies – circumstances in which they do are the exceptions and not the rule. The following account deals with the management of certain occupational condi tions where the occupational physician should be able to make a useful contribution, emphasizing those that are most common or that occur in a wide range of occupations. It also considers those relatively few and rare circumstances in which specific therapies in particular antidotes can be used to manage occupational disease such as poisoning. These include poisoning by anticholinesterases, cyanides and certain metals, methaemoglobinaemia and hydrofluoric acid burns.

Management of specific conditions resulting from exposure to hazardous substances

Occupational asthma and rhinitis

The mainstay of management of these conditions rests on the correct identification of the causative factors and on the appropriate preventive steps which are discussed in Chapters 3 and 5. Nevertheless, there are certain circumstances when specific therapy is indicated. These are the treatment of severe symptoms, temporary steps to treat milder symptoms while preventive steps are actively pursued, and the treatment of residual illness once all preventive steps have been implemented.

Occupational asthma, like asthma from other causes, can be a fatal disease. Isocyanates, reactive dyes and perhaps other agents have been responsible for preventable deaths in the workplace. Continuing exposure, the lack of appreciation of clinical features of deterioration and ignorance of the potential for worsening of symptoms in the hours after exposure has stopped are potential contributory factors. Medical and nursing staff at industrial sites where an asthma hazard exists must therefore be trained and equipped to deal with an asthmatic crisis by the administration of nebulized bronchodilators, say salbutamol or terbutaline, delivered ultrasonically or by oxygen from a cylinder. This may need to be followed by high concentration oxygen therapy. After the immediate emergency is over, two other important steps must be taken. An informed handover of clinical care to the general practitioner or to hospital medical staff supported by an explanation to the employee of the risk of deterioration is essential. Furthermore, the employee (and the manager) must be unequivocally advised against return to the particular job or to another with similar exposures until there has been clinical recovery and the physician and manager have taken all necessary steps to prevent a recurrence.

Case history 4.6

A 40 year-old process worker in the pharmaceutical industry presented to the occupational health centre complaining of shortness of breath. He was a nonsmoker and had worked in that industry for 22 years. A few days previously he had developed a cold which he could not shake off and which had gone to his chest. On examination he was clearly distressed with wheezing and other signs of bronchial narrowing. His FEV1/FVC was 1.8/3.9 litres. This improved after inhaled salbutamol to 2.6/5.4 litres. These values contrasted sharply with the results on routine health surveillance a year previously of 4.3/6.1 litres. Further enquiry revealed that for the previous week or two he had been working in a different part of the factory from his usual place because of the absence of a colleague. About 12 years previously he recollected having suffered from wheezy bronchitis when he had worked in that part of the plant. A provisional diagnosis of occupational asthma was made and after his symptoms were adequately relieved in the occupational health centre, he was given a detailed letter for his general practitioner and a bronchodilator inhaler, and driven home.

The occupational physician's awareness of the diagnosis, and the availability of adequate treatment options had permitted the man's symptoms to be rapidly and effectively relieved. It is not possible to predict the outcome had the treatment not been given on site. He almost certainly would have survived a journey to hospital without treatment, but may have become more distressed in the meantime. Not all cases of acute occupational asthma have made it to the hospital alive.

On return to work, arrangements had been made by the occupational physician for the employee to be recommenced in his usual location where he had been asymptomatic for at least 10 years. Serial peak expiratory flow rate (PEFR) measurements were commenced. A few days later he returned with the following note from his general practitioner 'this patient who did have some bronchospasm when he had a chest infection . . . is clinically well and his PEFR today is 610 litres/min which is well above the 95th centile for his height'. The worker refused further PEFR tests and further history-taking revealed that he was concerned about implications that a diagnosis of occupational asthma might have for his continuing employment.

Fear of the consequences that the diagnosis of an occupational disease may have upon employment, or ignorance of its manifestations can be serious impediments to both correct diagnosis and management. These points have been well illustrated by the above case. In spite of these difficulties the initial clinical management of this particular case was correct. Further medical management assumed that this was a sentinel case and a survey of the rest of the workforce was undertaken. This showed that there was a previously unrecognized asthma hazard and steps were taken to reduce the risk of this by containment, local exhaust ventilation and personal protective equipment. The occupational physician is sometimes faced with an awkward situation when an employee, for career advancement or for financial reasons insists that he is willing to tolerate work in an environment where exposure is such as to provoke symptoms of occupational asthma and/or rhinitis. Where there is a risk of anything but the mildest asthma or where it is envisaged that relevant exposure will continue indefinitely, there can be no compromise. A level of control adequate to abolish the occupational asthma must be insisted on, or failing that, a relocation of the employee. However, a very short term compromise between social factors and treatment of symptoms so long as they are mild may apply for example in a postgraduate student who develops laboratory animal allergy but who wishes to complete his project or in an industrial employee while control measures are implemented. Standard therapy for rhinitis and/or asthma, namely the use of antihistamines, beta agonists, corticosteroids or cromolyns as appropriate, would be prescribed by the employee's general practitioner in liaison with the occupational physician, who would closely monitor the situation.

Once exposure to an agent causing occupational asthma has ceased, some employees with this condition may have a persistence of their symptoms. In simple terms, exposure to the hazardous agent may have resulted in a syndrome clinically indistinguishable from 'intrinsic' or 'idiopathic' asthma. In these cases management of the asthma should be undertaken and continued in the same way as for asthma of other causes.

Angio-oedema

This is a very rare emergency in an industrial context. Nevertheless, severe anaphylactic reactions leading to angio-oedema could occur, for example, in a small proportion of individuals sensitized to laboratory animal allergens (see case history 4.2). It is false to assume that this rare but severe event is completely unpredictable. Affected workers often give a history of earlier milder episodes with urticaria and palpebral oedema. These heralds should be heeded. Moreover, a very small risk may be associated with vaccination.

In those workplaces where such risks apply, the appropriate therapeutic agents should be available for use by an occupational health professional. Essentially, these include ampoules containing 1 ml of 1:1,000 adrenaline to be administered intramuscularly and parenteral antihistamines, both of which can be expected to act quickly, as well as hydrocortisone which requires several hours to achieve a maximal effect and should not be given alone.

Occupational skin disease

Eczema/dermatitis is the commonest occupational skin disease that any physician will come across. As with asthma and rhinitis the principal element in the management of occupational dermatitis is avoidance of exposure to the causative agent and to any aggravating factors. Avoidance of exposure does not simply entail advice to wear gloves. The gloves or gauntlets should be adequate in their coverage and resistant to relevant physical damage and to the chemicals in use in the workplace. Thus, for example, ordinary rubber gloves do not provide adequate protection from many organic solvents. Care should also be taken that the gloves do not cause nor aggravate the dermatitis. The possibility of allergy to gloves should be considered when dermatitis does not resolve and tends to correspond initially to the area of the glove in its distribution. Moreover, any gloves may cause or aggravate dermatitis by irritation if the skin is weepy or sweaty when they are worn. In severe cases of dermatitis one may have to await substantial improvement before returning to work and then only wearing appropriate gloves. In some cases the wearing inside of cotton inserts which are replaced at least daily can reduce the risk of maceration from sweat and friction. The patient needs to be advised about possible irritants to avoid, whether occupational or otherwise, which while not necessarily causative could aggravate a dermatitis. These could include washing up liquids, shampoos and even soap. This can be a time-consuming task with limited retention of the advice by the patient. However, the involvement of an occupational health nurse and the provision of written advice such as an information sheet can help resolve both of these difficulties. Emollients such as emulsifying ointments and aqueous cream can be a useful adjunct to the treatment of irritant dermatitis associated with a dry skin especially if caused by defatting organic solvents or detergents. They should be applied liberally at least twice daily (just before and after a night's sleep) if it is not convenient to apply topical treatment during the working day. Creams and ointments, however, may make a wet weepy dermatitis worse. Barrier creams should be considered barriers only in name, since in most instances they provide no protective function at all and sometimes may even act as vehicles to promote the transport of harmful substances into the skin. However, some may have an emollient function or may assist hand cleaning. Topical corticosteroids may be necessary to assist in the resolution of occupational dermatitis as a supplement to, and not a substitute for cessation of exposure. They should be recommended in close liaison with the general practitioner.

It is best if the physician is familiar with one or two preparations and uses these. The rare but not extinct practice in some workplace medical centres of handing out topical corticosteroids without adequate assessment, protection from exposure or professional advice can only warrant serious criticism. It bears repeating that the management of occupational diseases should include assessment of the workplace and advice to prevent recurrence.

Case history 4.7

A pharmaceutical worker developed itching, redness and subsequently blistering of the fingers and back of the hand. At presentation in the occupational health department she had tense bullae, surrounded by inflamed skin. She was referred to hospital where de-roofing of the bullae was carried out aseptically. After several weeks she made a full functional and cosmetic recovery. History-taking and review of the process and the workplace showed that she had been handling a potent alkylating agent (mechlorethamine), while wearing black natural rubber gloves. The occupational physician found information that such gloves are permeable to this and similar agents, and advised that as well as a review of the workplaces, appropriate alternative gloves should be used.

In this case a detailed hazard assessment and preventive steps including the use of rubber gloves had been taken by the managing chemist and the safety officer. In spite of this, protection was not adequate and the occupational physician was able to make a useful contribution to the management of the problem.

Chemical asphyxiation

Contrary to popular belief, very few poisons can be treated by the use of specific antidotes. Indeed, even time-hallowed dogma on the use of various antidotes is now being called into question. The single most important step in the management of asphyxiation from whatever cause is removal of the victim to a place of safety and administration of oxygen in high concentration (see case history 4.5). Some special intoxications are worthy of further mention. In poisoning by cyanide (hydrogen cyanide or its salts) the mainstay of specific treatment used to be the binding of the cyanide to methaemoglobin produced by the administration of amyl nitrite by inhalation. Cobalt EDTA followed this treatment but this antidote is highly toxic and can kill the worker, especially if the diagnosis is mistaken. It should only be administered to an unconscious patient in whom cyanide poisoning has been proven, at least circumstantially, by environmental measurement. Intravenous administration must be slow and cautious and may result in angio-oedema. A more recently advocated treatment which is safer and might be equally effective is the intravenous administration of hydroxocobalamin, which combines with cyanide to form cyanocobalamin. Poisoning with other chemical asphyxiants such as carbon monoxide (e.g. from incomplete combustion) or hydrogen sulphide (e.g. from decomposition of sewage) should likewise be treated with high concentration oxygen. In severe cases, urgent transfer to a hyperbaric centre should be considered.

Methaemoglobinaemia can result from exposure by inhalation or by splash to agents such as aniline or nitrobenzene. For reasons which are poorly understood the electronic configuration of the iron in haem changes and the haemoglobin is converted to methaemoglobin which is incapable of carrying oxygen. This substance is more blue in colour than normal haemoglobin and this contributes to the clinical cyanosis. Oxygen and rest are very important in the treatment, besides rigorous decontamination. The specific antidote for symptomatic cases consists of methylene blue administered slowly intravenously, although ascorbic acid (Vitamin C) has also been employed.

Irritant gases

Irritant chemicals, such as chlorine and ammonia, and even the less irritant nitrogen dioxide, may cause acute pulmonary oedema, within hours of exposure, and a delayed obliterative bronchiolitis, which may present with breathlessness some weeks after the exposure. The most common industrial gassings are due to chlorine, in the chemical industry and many other workplaces where it is used as a bleach or disinfectant. It even causes problems occasionally in swimming pools and in domestic cleaning where hypochlorites may inadvertently be mixed with acids. Nitrogen dioxide may be generated in silos, by welding and by combustion of cellulose. Many other toxic and irritant gases may be encountered in industry, and occupational physicians should always keep an eye open for places where they could be liberated or accumulated.

Case history 4.8

A 48 year-old man was employed by a local authority as a chargehand at a sewage pumping station. His duties included climbing down into an open sewage channel in the building to scrub down its walls with a brush. There was usually only a small stream of soiled water running at the bottom of this channel. On one occasion, whilst doing this job he noticed that the smell was even more unpleasant than usual. Since workers doing this sort of work learn to tolerate awful smells he continued scrubbing until he started to cough and became short of breath. He also felt faint, but managed to climb out of the channel before losing consciousness. His workmate, who had been out, fortunately came back at this moment, dragged him out of the building and administered oxygen. He was taken to hospital with an acute toxic pneumonitis from which he eventually made a full recovery. Analysis of this gas in the pumping station and subsequent investigation showed that there had been an illegal disposal of chemicals by a large factory into the sewage system the previous night probably resulting in the release of hydrogen sulphide. This had made its way through the pipes to the station by the time the patient had started work.

This patient was fortunate. Many people gassed in tanks or culverts never make it out, and sometimes their workmates also die trying to rescue them. His pulmonary oedema settled in hospital with oxygen and corticosteroids.

In the first aid treatment of exposure to these substances, the rescuers having first ascertained their own safety, using breathing apparatus if necessary, must then remove the victim and administer oxygen in high concentration. Some advocate the use of inhaled corticosteroids in the workplace when exposure to irritant gases has occurred. This policy runs the risk of being unnecessary in a number of cases and inadequate in the rest. If there has been a non-trivial exposure to an irritant gas that could lead to pulmonary oedema, the best counsel is for the worker to be hospitalized, for full assessment. In most serious cases it is wise to give systemic corticosteroids at this stage as there is anecdotal evidence of their effectiveness.

Pesticide intoxications

Many pesticides contain organophosphates or carbamates, potent cholinesterase inhibitors. Occupational exposure may take place through inhalation of mists generated by spraying or through eye or skin absorption. Warm weather makes it less likely that the worker will wear adequate protection, as well as aggravating the physiological consequences of exposure. The symptoms and signs are those of uninhibited acetylcholine-mediated neurotransmission. They range from headaches, nausea, lassitude and visual disturbance, through lacrimation, salivation, abdominal cramp, vomiting, bradycardia and tremors, to pulmonary oedema, convulsions, coma and death. When this type of poisoning is suspected, a blood sample should be taken for cholinesterase assay even if treatment has to be instituted rapidly. The worker, as in many other intoxications where skin contamination is likely, must be stripped and washed thoroughly with soap and water. The attendants must have due regard for their own safety during this procedure. Secretions should be cleared and oxygen administered if necessary. Intravenous atropine in doses substantially higher than the ordinary therapeutic range may need to be administered repeatedly. This drug blocks the cholinergic muscarinic receptors but does not deal with the underlying problem. Tachycardia and pupillary dilatation indicate adequate atropinization. Further management of severe organophosphate (but not carbamate) poisoning includes early administration of intravenous pralidoxime to reactivate the cholinesterase.

Other poisonings – the role of poisons centres

National and regional poisons centres have a very important role to play in the management of occupational intoxications. Although they deal most commonly with poisonings by therapeutic substances and household agents, they can contribute in an advisory capacity or by clinical management of cases of industrial poisoning. They are usually accessed by telephone and some can be interrogated electronically.

Chemical burns

Emergency management of chemical burns starts essentially with prolonged (more than 15 minutes) irrigation with tap water. Any of the worker's clothes which could have been contaminated should be gently stripped. If one hazardous agent is to be singled out as a special example then it probably should be hydrofluoric acid. This dangerous substance is more ubiquitous than one may at first imagine, as for example its use in etching of glass for labelling and security reasons. It is rapidly corrosive to the skin, other soft tissues and bone. If exposure is substantial it may cause systemic upset through hypocalcaemia produced by the binding of calcium to the fluoride ions. Treatment locally should include the liberal irrigation with calcium gluconate solution, and in hospital intravenous calcium gluconate may be needed to combat the hypocalcaemia. Many chemical burns may need the early involvement of plastic surgeons in case skin grafting should prove necessary.

The eye is of course particularly sensitive to chemical burns and substances such as alkalis – which are present in domestic dishwasher powders and oven cleaning agents and not only in 'heavy industry' – as well as acids, can inflict terrible damage. All such injuries should be thoroughly irrigated in the workplace and where there is any doubt at all about residual harm to the eye, the employee should be referred for specialist examination, including fluorescein instillation, using a slit lamp.

Management of conditions resulting from exposure to physical agents

Radiation

There are various aspects of the management of certain peculiarly occupational physical exposures which deserve attention. Exposure to ionizing radiation without adequate safeguards can be a serious medical emergency. An occupational physician facing such a prospect should either have been adequately trained beforehand or at least be aware of the need to urgently seek expert advice. The Radiation Protection Adviser (RPA) has an important function in assessing the risk of exposure to radiation and in giving advice on its control. The RPA is responsible for monitoring radiation at source and for organizing personal dosimetry through film badges worn on clothing, thermoluminescent dosimeters attached to extremities or direct reading electrometers. The RPA gives advice about segregation, containment, handling and disposal of radioactive materials. The RPA, however, can also help in a retrospective estimate of radiation exposure from a review of the circumstances which have led to it. The physician has a role to play in biological dosimetry in the case of substantial whole body radiation; an appropriate blood sample must be taken early for a white cell count and lymphocyte culture for chromosome analysis, since these indices correlate well with exposure to ionizing radiation at relatively high doses of over-exposure.

The acute hazards of non-ionizing radiation to the skin have been ex-emplified in case history 2.3. The eye is very sensitive to light injury, to varying degrees dependent on wavelength and intensity, but 'Arc eye' is a classical example of corneal injury caused by ultraviolet light from arc welding. There may be a latent period of up to one day before symptoms of keratitis develop. It is treated symptomatically but cessation of further uncontrolled exposure is essential.

Thermal hazards

In most of today's occupations, the risks of thermal hazards are generally small. Thus in hot humid kitchens, particularly in workers of a small physique, there is a risk of faints. This is especially so among new employees, who may be over- zealous and not yet acclimatized. Usually simple environmental steps such as improvement in ventilation, task rotation, wearing appropriate clothing and acclimatization are enough to prevent recurrence. Fluid and salt replenishment should be encouraged.

More prolonged exposure to heat, indoors or outdoors can result in heat stress or heat exhaustion. The patient is unwell and may feel faint or nauseated, or experience cramps, while thermoregulation and hence sweating is maintained. Simple common sense measures as outlined above are usually adequate, but if the condition is not recognized and managed appropriately it may lead to heat stroke.

Heat stroke (hyperpyrexia) is a medical emergency with a very high mortal-ity if not recognized early and treated vigorously. It is characterized by a rise in core body temperature above 40 °C due to the failure of the thermoregulatory mechanism; in the absence of sweating there is tissue damage notably to the liver, kidneys and brain. Thus the patient may be comatose or delirious, and may even have seizures. The afflicted worker must be removed urgently from the hot environment, vigorously cooled by wetting and by measures to increase evaporation, together with general supportive measures; an intravenous infusion should be instituted pending transfer to intensive care. Fortunately, this is a rare condition in industry in temperate climates although it still occurs from time to time, especially in the armed forces on training exercises. In any particular case the occupational physician must assess the circumstances giving rise to these health effects and give advice on measures to prevent recurrence. This should include improvements in the general environment, provision of appropriate clothing, information and instruction about the risks, changes in work practices and removal of particularly susceptible individuals.

Hypothermia can arise occupationally when the worker is immersed in water or exposed to cold air; for a given environmental temperature the former is more rapid in onset than the latter. However, in conditions which are windy, the chilling effect of the wind especially in a wet, exhausted and inadequately protected subject, is often underestimated. It is very important for the physician to be aware of the risks and not to miss the diagnosis. The core temperature should be measured, hypothermia being diagnosed usually if it is less than 35 °C. The absence of shivering can be a feature of the seriousness of the condition and may be followed by delirium, coma and death. First aid management should start with the application of thermal blankets but may go on to intravenous infusion and warming with water not exceeding 40 °C until the core temperature reaches 35 °C. As with hyperpyrexia, hypothermia is a medical emergency warranting specialist management of such complications as acid base imbalance. In severe cases when vital signs are absent resuscitation attempts should be prolonged, as the low body temperature may protect the brain and other organs from irreversible hypoxic damage for much longer than in a normothermic cardiac arrest.

Pressure hazards

Workers exposed to raised ambient air pressures as in diving, caisson work, or compressed air tunnelling, or reduced pressures as in flying are usually protected by specialist medical advice and support. Nevertheless, the generalist should be aware of the risks that may be associated with an abnormal environmental pressure so that specialist advice can be sought in a preventive context, and so that the clinical manifestations after a pressure related event can be recognized early. Complaints of any symptoms such as headache, nausea, vertigo, limb pain or pareses after work in abnormal pressure environments must therefore be treated seriously and referred immediately to the nearest hyperbaric facility.

Management of exposure to infectious agents

Accidental exposure to infectious agents warranting specific intervention occurs most frequently in health care or laboratory contexts but may also be encountered in other situations involving the emergency services or local authority employees. As in all the previously mentioned circumstances, a good history with pertinent questions is essential to assess exposure. Having assessed the risk of transmission of infection following exposure and determined that active treatment is warranted this can follow either of two routes: immunization or drug treatment. Post-event immunization against such conditions as tetanus and tuberculosis are well covered in non-occupational texts but management of potential viral exposure incidents deserves special mention.

Case history 4.9

An operating theatre attendant in a general hospital injured himself with a suture needle while clearing up after an operating session. He reported to the casualty department where the doctor did not take a vaccination history nor seek to enquire about the patient on whom the needle could have been used. The attendant had his wound cleaned and was given tetanus toxoid in the casualty department, reassured and sent away. Later when speaking to a better informed colleague he was asked whether he had been protected against Hepatitis B and when he answered negatively it was suggested that he refer himself to the occupational health department.

Case history 4.10

A depressive patient in a psychiatric institution committed suicide by throwing himself from a window several floors up. A psychiatric nurse attempted to administer mouth-to-mouth resuscitation and contaminated her mouth with blood from the patient's facial injuries as a result. She sought the advice of a trainee psychiatrist at the scene who reassured her that the acids in her stomach would destroy any organism, so she need not be unduly worried. However she had lingering doubts and the next day she presented to the occupational health department seeking further advice.

In both the above cases a woefully inadequate risk assessment was carried out by the doctors involved. Luckily neither of the two exposed staff developed Hepatitis B, and both of them were later offered and given Hepatitis B vaccination by the occupational health service. The occupational physician took steps to inform and educate staff at the two hospitals concerned. This consisted of discussing and agreeing policy with the senior staff, providing this information in induction courses and circulars to staff and publicizing it by means of posters; thus it is now most unlikely that junior medical staff there would give similar inadequate advice.

Where an immunologically unprotected worker sustains a needlestick or similar injury breaching the skin, or else a splash to a mucous membrane or inflamed skin with blood which is not known nor demonstrated to be free from Hepatitis B virus, immunization is appropriate. The conventional treatment consists of the administration of Hepatitis B hyperimmune gamma globulin intramuscularly in a dose of 500 units. This should be given as soon as possible after the exposure and in any event within 2 days together with the commencement of active immunization with Hepatitis B vaccine. Other management such as wound toilet may be necessary, although in case history 4.9 the chances of exposure to tetanus spores in an operating theatre must have been rather remote! Drug therapy may be needed in the post-event prophylaxis of other exposures to infectious agents, as exemplified in the next case history.

Case history 4.11

A medical registrar was summoned urgently to a patient suffering from systemic lupus erythematosus who was on treatment with high dose steroids and who had been readmitted severely shocked. Very shortly after the doctor's arrival the patient sustained a cardiac arrest. Attempts at resuscitation including mouth-to-mouth respiration were unsuccessful. The next day, blood cultures from samples taken during the failed resuscitation attempt showed a heavy growth of Neisseria meningitidis. The registrar sought advice and was administered, uneventfully, 600 mg of rifampicin orally twice daily for two days.

While the above post-event prophylaxis is uncontroversial, there is considerable uncertainty and debate on the management of possible exposure to HIV, the causative agent of acquired immune deficiency syndrome – AIDS. This situation is illustrated by case history 4.12.

Case history 4.12

A nurse in a casualty department was undressing a semi-comatose young man, who was suspected of being a drug addict. While removing his jacket, she pricked her finger on a needle in his pocket. This turned out to be attached to a syringe which contained blood from a recent self-injection and the needle had penetrated quite deeply. At the time of the incident, the hospital was just finalizing its policy for the management of such problems. The wound was encouraged to bleed, blood was taken from the patient for subsequent testing for Hepatitis B and HIV antigen (the patient had already said he was HIV positive) and the nurse was immediately given a booster dose of Hepatitis B vaccine, having previously had a course with a good antibody response. According to the new policy, she was seen and counselled within one hour by the infectious diseases consultant and given zidovudine (Syn AZT: azidothymidine) intravenously. On further follow-up, with her informed consent, the HIV status was monitored and fortunately she did not become positive.

This was an unusually clear-cut case, where there was little doubt that a risk of infection existed. It has been estimated that the risk in such circumstances is about 5 per cent for Hepatitis B and about 10 times less for HIV. The prevention and post-injury management of Hepatitis B risk is straightforward since active and passive immunization is readily available. But the management of HIV exposure is much more problematic. In this case, the physician's first step is to assess the problem, by trying to determine the likelihood of infection of the source although this can present ethical problems discussed below. The worker should be counselled about the risks and consequences of infection, and the implications of testing. Thus insurance firms tend to look adversely at applicants who have had a test for HIV antibody undertaken, regardless of the reason for this or the outcome. A suitable compromise may be merely to take serum on presentation and after an interval of a few months and store it, only to be tested with the worker's consent at a later date if clinically indicated. Finally the circumstances of the case must be reviewed in consultation with the manager to take action to prevent future episodes by introducing appropriate policies, information and changes in work practices.

As in the above case, the antiviral drug zidovudine has been administered by some physicians to health care workers after needlestick or similar injuries from HIV positive sources. The course is started within an hour of the incident and up to 2 g are given daily in divided doses for 4–6 weeks. There is no evidence in humans that this line of action reduces the risk of seroconversion and indeed there are case reports where such a protocol has manifestly failed to protect individual employees. Moreover the drug in question may have severe side effects including bone marrow depression. On the balance of current evidence, the routine use of AZT for the post-event prophylaxis of HIV infection is not recommended except perhaps for large inoculums of proven HIV positive blood. The reader is advised to keep up with the publications which will continue to appear on this subject for up-to-date advice. In any case careful documentation of the event and follow up is essential. The exposed employee should be advised to have serum stored in order to keep the option open for testing at a later date if so counselled and agreed. If voluntary reporting schemes or research projects are in progress the physician should be encouraged to participate in the data collection for these activities.

Special ethical dilemmas can arise when attempting to determine the risks of infectious exposure of employees. While many physicians responsible for the care of patients who may have been the source of body fluids to which a health care employee has been exposed will disclose risk factors or the results of investigations (such as Hepatitis B status) at the request of a physician caring for the employee, this extent of cooperation is not always universal. Furthermore, the current ethical consensus in respect of HIV infection is that it is not acceptable for a patient to be tested without full informed consent accompanied by appropriate counselling. This requirement is generally held to be paramount and therefore to take precedence over assessing the risk to employees. Although it appears incongruent with other policies and practices in regard to occupational health risk assessment, it has at present to be respected.

Serious ethical problems may also arise when employees in certain occupations may be carriers of Hepatitis B and HIV. In the vast majority of occupational contexts such infection in itself has no implications for fitness for work, unless the consequent physical impairment is such as to present a disability in undertaking tasks effectively or safely. However in occupations such as invasive surgery, dentistry, vascular catheterization, extra corporeal perfusion (in theatres or in renal support units) and obstetric procedures during which bleeding can occur, there is a small, but finite, risk of infection with Hepatitis B or HIV being transmitted from employees to the patients they care for. Various professional bodies have produced ethical guidance on this as have advisers to the British Department of Health. Thus for example the recommendation of the Expert Advisory Group on Aids is that 'health care workers who have or suspect they are infected with HIV must seek expert advice on whether there is need to limit or alter their work practice'. It must also not be forgotten that employees have wide responsibilities, under Health and Safety at work legislation, to reduce the risks to others and to cooperate with employers in ensuring health and safety. Employees engaged in jobs such as those mentioned above must seek the advice of the occupational health physician if they know or suspect that they might be infected with Hepatitis B or HIV. Full counselling on the social, domestic and occupational implications of possible infection must precede testing. The doctor should if possible be in a position to confirm the employer's commitment to safeguard the confidentiality and employment of employees; ideally this matter should have been discussed and a policy agreed with management before the first case occurs. Unless these reassurances are explicit, honoured and believed, employees will be very reluctant to come forward for help and advice in spite of all the pronouncements of various professional and other bodies. Clinical investigations can help confirm or estimate some aspects of the risk of transmission; thus in employees who have a history of Hepatitis B (HBsAg positive) or who have apparently not responded to Hepatitis B vaccination, serological measures of the 'e' antigen (HBeAg) are an index of high infectivity if positive. In some cases investigation may indicate the possible value of treatment, for example with interferon.

Once the risk of transmitting infection has been thoroughly assessed on an individual basis by an occupational physician, often in conjunction with another relevant specialist, the employee and the employer should be advised about it and consideration given to appropriate redeployment.

Reporting of occupational disease and injury

Legislation regarding occupational disease has three limbs, dealing with its prevention, compensation for sufferers and reporting of cases. The third of these is little known to doctors, and is often neglected. Reporting is not a mere vexation imposed by the legislators, but fulfils certain functions:

- It provides an opportunity for the episode and compliance with the law to be investigated.
- It should lead to steps for the prevention of similar episodes locally.
- It contributes to national data for assessing the size of the problem and the effectiveness of preventing legislation.
- It permits the establishment of better priorities and targets for national preventive strategies.

In the United Kingdom the mainstay of the legal requirement for reporting occupational ill-health or injury consists of the Reporting of Injuries, Diseases and Dangerous Occurrences Regulations (RIDDOR). These place the responsibility for reporting squarely on the employer's shoulders. However, in the case of occupational diseases, the employer has to act on a diagnosis provided by a doctor (and not necessarily an occupational physician). The main reportable occupational diseases under these regulations (see Appendix 1) include poisoning by various chemical agents such as benzene and lead, certain skin diseases (but not the commonest one, eczema/dermatitis), asthma and other respiratory diseases and various cancers (which are also prescribed – see below, page 99). The provisions include the reporting of so-called vibration white finger but not occupational deafness – a much commoner condition, nor of tenosynovitis or other allied musculoskeletal conditions. Indeed the paradox of these regulations is the absence of a requirement to report what are perhaps the three commonest categories of occupational organic disease in the UK, deafness, musculoskeletal problems and dermatitis. Under the regulations, reportable injuries include fractures of any bones except for those in the foot or hand, amputations, loss of sight and penetration injury or burns to the eye. Many other injuries are specified including any injury causing incapacity for normal work (not necessarily sickness absence) for more than 3 days (see Chapter 6).

It has to be recognized that even for the categories of disease and injury which are reportable there is evidence of considerable under-reporting. The occupational physician should take steps to bridge this gap. Thus employers should be explicitly advised in writing when a reportable injury or disease is encountered by the physician. If the employee does not consent to this, then it is recommended that the physician makes a direct confidential approach to the Health and Safety Executive, explaining the employee's concerns as well as the facts of the case.

In addition to the legal responsibilities for reporting, there are various voluntary schemes, participation in which is to be encouraged. The purposes of such schemes may differ from those of statutory ones, for example to provide information which may be used for research into causes, management and prevention of disease. In the UK the best known is SWORD (surveillance of work related and occupational respiratory disease). This involves regular reporting by occupational physicians and chest physicians of a wide range of cases of respiratory disease which could be work related. The list is by no means limited to those conditions which are reportable, or prescribed by law and has confirmed the impression of under-reporting of many of these diseases. Occupational and other relevant physicians are strongly encouraged to participate in this and similar schemes such as those addressing urothelial tumours, skin diseases and blood diseases.

Compensation

In most cases money is a poor substitute for the suffering and shortening of life caused by disease to the patient, or for bereavement by relatives. Nevertheless, compensation is a mechanism to help provide for lost earnings and other damages. It is important that the physician is aware of the mechanism for awarding compensation for occupational disease. In the UK compensation, broadly speaking, falls into two categories – industrial injuries benefits from the state through the Department of Social Security and compensation from the employer or insurer through common law civil litigation.

Industrial injuries benefits

Case history 4.13

A baker aged 60 working in a hospital suffered from progressively worsening bronchial asthma, needing treatment with beta adrenergic and anti-cholinergic bronchodilators as well as corticosteroids. He gave no history of asthma in childhood or adolescence, the asthmatic symptoms having started after he began work as a baker. They remitted when he had a spell away from baking but returned when he resumed this trade latterly with the Health Service. He also had a history of rhinitis with polyps and had had about five nasal polypectomies. His symptoms became so severe that he could no longer cope with his work. He had never been made aware that his work could cause such symptoms but the history was strongly suggestive of occupational asthma and a visit to his workplace showed substantial exposure to airborne flour. Apparently, previous doctors had not considered the possibility that his symptoms could be occupational. He was given a peak flow meter with instructions for self-monitoring, but the readings did not conclusively show a work related pattern; after several years of symptoms and with multiple therapy, this was not surprising. He proved to have a very poor exercise tolerance which did not improve after sickness absence, but even if there had been an improvement, there was no early prospect of the hospital bakery reducing his exposure to flour dust substantially.

What was the occupational physician to do? Sadly premature retirement on grounds of ill-health was the only option since no prospects of relocation to another sedentary job for which he might be fit were found. He might in fact have been short changed by the Health Service twice – as an employee he had not had adequate information and protection, and as a patient the possible relation between his symptoms and his work had gone unrecognized until late in his condition.

What compensation could be available? While some doctors and lay people erroneously believe that the role of the Department of Social Security is to guard the treasury and avoid paying out compensation if at all possible, the reality is rather different. The process is simple, as follows:

- The doctor making the diagnosis checks that the patient has been employed in a prescribed occupation (see Appendix 1), and that there is therefore a likelihood that he or she will be eligible for benefits.
- The patient is advised to make a claim at the Department of Social Security for industrial injury (or in this case, pneumoconiosis) benefits. This is done by filling in a form.
- The patient is told that the process involves an insurance official at the Department checking that he or she was employed in a prescribed occupation and then referring him or her to a doctor for diagnosis and assessment of disablement.
- The doctors employed by the Department, in this case in the Medical Boarding Centre (Respiratory Diseases), will generally see the patient and, often after consultation with the specialist involved or obtaining lung function tests, determine the diagnosis and assess disability in terms of 'loss of faculty'. This clinical assessment, based on history, examination and special tests, compares the individual to another of the same age and sex, taking account of his job.
- A loss of faculty of, say, 50 per cent is communicated to the insurance office, who will generally arrange payment of a pension equal to 50 per cent of the maximum sum voted each year by Parliament. A lump sum is occasionally paid instead of pension.
- The patient will often be reviewed by the Department's doctors from time to time.

The conclusion of the Department may not always be that of the patient or the patient's doctor. For example, diffuse pleural fibrosis or lung cancer in the presence of asbestosis attract benefits, while pleural plaques or lung cancer in an ex-asbestos worker with no fibrosis do not. Where the patient's claim is turned down, there is an appeals procedure through an independent panel, the Medical Appeals Tribunal.

The list of prescribed diseases and occupations is under regular review by the independent Industrial Injuries Advisory Council. Any doctor who believes that an occupational disease should be on the list is able to write with the evidence and ask for the matter to be considered. In general the rule is that the disease must be a specific risk of the occupation and not a general risk of other people, thus allowing the connection between cause and effect to be made clinically in an individual.

Compensation through common law

There are some very important differences between compensation obtained through Social Security legislation and that obtained in a court of law by a civil action against an employer or ex-employer. In both instances there has to be good evidence of occupational disease and relevant exposure, and a physician with appropriate training may be able to give a good opinion about these points. However, additionally, for a civil case to succeed, the court must be satisfied that the employer ought to have known about the risks and could and should have done more to prevent them in the light of knowledge at the time; that is, the employer was negligent. The employer in turn may seek to prove that the injured worker was negligent in not taking steps to prevent the disease, that the disease occurred as a consequence of unforeseeable individual susceptibility, or indeed that the worker does not have the disease in question or is suffering little or no real disability. Some of these matters are beyond the area of expertise of many doctors, who should therefore usually confine themselves to matters of diagnosis, level of disability and prognosis. Since the case is heard by a judge and argued by lawyers, the process is both costly and lengthy, and the outcome is never certain. Many cases are settled out of court by a bargaining process, but the possibility that the doctor will be cross-examined should give pause to the wary – only experts should write expert reports! Because of the complexities of the legal process, doctors should be cautious before suggesting that the patient embarks on a time-consuming, expensive and sometimes distressing legal action. If the diagnosis is reasonably secure (in court it is decided on the basis of the balance of probabilities – more likely than not) and negligence is possible, the worker should be referred to his trade union or a lawyer.

Practically anything written by a physician may be the subject of 'discovery' i.e. may be sought by a legal process, reviewed by solicitors and scrutinized publicly in a court of law. An important exception is a report written by a physician specifically for the purpose of advising a lawyer in a case of litigation. However since such a report is often by its very nature intended to help pursue or defend a claim it is often challenged in a court of law. It therefore follows that a physician must at all times exercise the highest standard of care and keep adequate and accurate written records. Thus all consultations should explicitly state the reason, relevant symptomatic and objective findings, the diagnostic and occupational implications, relevant advice imparted and to whom (see Chapter 10). A medicolegal report should be more detailed, with certain added elements. Thus it should contain a short statement of the credentials, i.e. qualifications, relevant experience and employment status of the physician making the report. It should state why the report was commissioned and by whom. The written informed consent of the worker for this purpose must be obtained and appended. After basic personal and social details a detailed occupational, symptomatic and if appropriate, past and family history is recorded. If the information comes from sources other than the patient, its respective origins should be defined. Physical examination is important not merely to the extent that in ordinary medical practice it may establish a diagnosis but also to corroborate (to the limited extent to which this may be possible) the historical assessment. The results of relevant investigations of the patient or of the workplace together with information regarding their source should follow. Care must be taken to explain all of this in 'lay' terms so that lawyers and the court can understand it easily. An opinion on the diagnosis should follow together with an interpretation of the likely causative or contributory factors. The prognosis, expressed principally in terms of health risk, occupational and social handicaps should follow. Any factors which could have influenced the outcome or could do so at a later date should be stated. An indication of the level of certainty with which the respective conclusions are reached, (again remembering that the legal test is the balance of probabilities) if necessary backed up by reasoned argument, is important.

In writing an expert's report the doctor should endeavour to answer all the questions posed by the lawyer, but should not draw conclusions which cannot be justified. However, the report should address all points which appear to be relevant to the issue even if they have not all been raised in the referring lawyer's questions. A useful attitude is to attempt to overlook the source of request for the report and to respond to it in a thoroughly professional and impartial manner, believing (as is usually the case) that what the lawyer wants is an expert view of the truth rather than poorly justified support for the client's case.

5

Prevention of occupational disease

Summary

The prevention of occupational disease takes the doctor into relatively un-familiar territory. This chapter describes the principles of the disciplines that make the largest contribution to ensuring workplace safety, ergonomics and occupational hygiene. Ergonomics is concerned primarily with interactions between man and the physical and psychological environment at work, while occupational hygiene is concerned mainly with measurement and control of harmful substances in the workplace. Some knowledge of ergonomics is helpful to doctors working in industry, both as an aid to diagnosis and also to help in the planning of measures to prevent injury and psychological ill-health. Similarly, an understanding of occupational hygiene allows doctors to give sensible advice on measures to protect workers from harmful substances.

The law puts an obligation on employers to take all reasonably practicable measures to ensure the health and safety of their employees. The workings of the relevant legislation are described in this chapter, as is the value as a source of advice of the Health and Safety Executive and its medical arm, the Employment Medical Advisory Service. Finally, the chapter mentions the role of selection of appropriate workers, as much to question the value of pre-employment screening as to promote it, but stresses the importance of education of workers and management in health and safety issues.

Introduction

In principle, all occupational injury and disease is preventable, and it is the business of the occupational physician to urge management as far as possible in this direction. While many managers are sympathetic to this endeavour and very few are careless of the welfare of their workers, their primary role is to make a profit or, at the least, to achieve a set financial target. It is a part of managerial decision-making to balance the cost of a particular decision against the likely benefits to the company. When it comes to deciding on measures to prevent ill-health, the equation becomes one of balancing the costs against the risk of occurrence. Prevention will only be implemented if it has a price tag which is reasonable when compared to the perceived benefits.

What then is the doctor's role? An important aspect involves the diagnosis and management of occupational disease, as outlined in Chapters 3 and 4. Since most workplaces do not have access to an occupational health service, the general practitioner or the hospital specialist is often the first person to suspect occupational disease. That doctor is therefore able, by taking appropriate action, to prevent similar conditions occurring in other workers. Where the company or organization does have access to an occupational health service, preventive measures may be taken at an earlier stage, before ill-health has occurred, if the doctor or nurse is aware of the possibility of risk and able to persuade managers to take appropriate action. Management of risk involves its assessment, planning of action to reduce it, implementation of the plan, and evaluation of the plan's success, just as management of disease requires clinical assessment, planning and administering treatment and follow-up. This simple logical approach is the basis of all preventive action in the workplace. The identification and assessment processes frequently require experience with a particular industry and with appropriate instruments for monitoring chemical and physical hazards. Some problems may be simple to resolve; others may require extensive and costly changes in plant structure and manufacturing/production process. Selection of appropriate working methods and good design of the workplace and working practices are the best solutions to any problem of workplace ill-health, but they often pose the greatest technical challenges to engineer and plant manager alike.

Preventive occupational medicine takes the physician into unfamiliar territory. Most doctors learn something in medical school of the important roles played in disease prevention by improvements in social factors such as housing, sanitation and employment opportunities, matters that we often take rather for granted until we are reminded of their importance by a visit to the Third World. Occupational ill health is prevented in an analogous manner, namely by the improvement of relevant factors in the workplace. Proper design of jobs and of the place where work is done will do much to prevent injury and accident – this is the business of the disciplines of ergonomics and safety management. Careful control of substances or physical factors that impose a risk on workers is the business of occupational hygiene. These two disciplines operate within a legislative framework, which defines the duties and responsibilities of managers and workers within the workplace. The physician concerned with workplace problems needs to know something of ergonomics, occupational hygiene, and health and safety law. In addition, in some areas of occupational medicine, immunization of workers may play a part in prevention, while in all cases training and education of workers and managers is important.

It will be noted that the emphasis of this chapter is on prevention by making the workplace safe. This should not be a surprise, but it is a fact that many managers erroneously believe that prevention should be based rather on selection of the superfit or disease-resistant at pre-employment examination. This is, of course, a misconception that flies in the face of efforts of doctors and others to rehabilitate less than fully fit people into the working population. Nevertheless, pre-employment selection of appropriate people for certain types of work is sometimes necessary, and this is also discussed in this chapter.

Ergonomics

Ergonomics is concerned with the interaction between the worker and the job. The simplest definition of ergonomics is 'the science of making the job fit the worker'; another is 'the application of human sciences to the optimization of people's working environment'. Ergonomics seeks to improve the match between the job and man's physical abilities, information handling and workload capacities. The subject is synonymous with 'human factors engineering', a term used in North America. Its fundamental importance is recognized in the International Labour Organization, which defines ergonomics as 'the application of the human biological sciences in conjunction with the engineering sciences to the worker and his working environment, so as to obtain maximum satisfaction for the worker which at the same time enhances productivity'. This definition emphasizes the important triad of ergonomic elements: comfort, health, and productivity.

Thus ergonomics seeks to adapt work to human physical and psychological capabilities and limitations. In seeking this goal, it draws on many disciplines including anatomy, physiology, psychology, sociology, physics, and engineering.

The value of ergonomics is easily understood by anyone who has tried to do a job using the wrong tools. The increased difficulty causes the job to take longer, leading to frustration and loss of temper. This in turn leads to use of excessive force and increases the risk of a slip of the hand and injury. In the wider world of industry and commerce, such problems arising from poor design of jobs, machines or workplaces may lead to large-scale inefficiencies, risk taking, increase in accidents and 'near-misses', and increases in absenteeism related to dissatisfaction with the job. The doctor working in industry, equipped with an understanding of ergonomic principles, is in a position to understand problems arising from interactions between people and their work, to plan solutions to such problems, and to help ensure that equipment is used safely and effectively. Knowledge of ergonomics may be of diagnostic value, for example in the investigation of musculo-skeletal disease, of aid in management, as in rehabilitating someone with back pain, and helpful as an adjunct to other preventive measures. For example, personal protective equipment will not generally be used unless it is acceptable to employees, by fitting comfortably and not interfering unduly with the task for which it is needed.

Case history 5.1

It was noted during a workplace visit that men working on coal silos were not wearing their safety harnesses. Failure to wear such equipment in the past had resulted in fatalities when workers had fallen and drowned or been crushed in the machine. The men said that the equipment was difficult to wear, and in any case did not work properly. A study was planned in which workers were presented with the various types of safety harness available, asked to put them on and were then hoisted up by a rope attached to a pulley. The results (Fig. 5.1) were revealing, most men having great difficulty donning the equipment, and often doing it incorrectly so that they slipped through or got caught in awkward positions.

The lesson of this simple experiment is that protective equipment needs to be designed with the user in mind. In this case, new designs of harness were necessary, and the manufacturer needed to test these on a panel of relatively unsophisticated workers before releasing them on the market. In any situation when people interact with machines or equipment, the application of ergonomics can prevent later dangerous and perhaps fatal consequences.

Some of the tasks of ergonomics are to achieve optimal working conditions by seeking to reduce excessive workload; to improve working postures; and to facilitate cognitive and psychomotor functions in the handling of working instruments, including avoidance of unnecessary recall of information and the appropriate placement of workers. Ergonomics is best employed *de novo* in designing the job. By designing tasks with human needs clearly in focus much can be done to prevent problems before they arise.

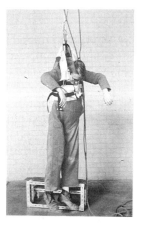

Fig. 5.1 Consequence of inadequate design of safety harness and training in its use

The role of ergonomics in occupational medicine

Ergonomics is almost unique in that it holds hope not only of reducing risk of injury and accident, but also of increasing productivity. By carefully designing a workplace or a job, the worker may be both safer and more effective in the task. The role of ergonomics, therefore, should be relatively easy to sell to managers, as a cost-effective means of improving safety.

Case history 5.2

A large and very expensive coalmining machine was designed to extract coal efficiently in difficult conditions underground. The engineering design was complex, but solutions were found and the machine was introduced into the workplace. However, the seat for the driver had been positioned in such a way that he was unable to see the drilling head when it was in action, thus requiring the use of an additional man as guide. The driver frequently had to stop the machine in order to stand up to see what he was doing. This failure to consider the sightlines of the operator was a fundamental design fault which cost money – in the need to employ another man and in the inefficiency of a stop-start operation. However, from a medical point of view, it also led to risk of accidents such as injury to the spotter by the machine itself or to the driver from frequent awkward movements. This latter problem was compounded by many other design faults in the layout and spacing of controls. As an example to designers, the ergonomist investigating this machine redesigned a man to fit easily into the machine and operate it (Fig. 5.2)!

In this example the problem was insoluble because of the investment already made in the machine. However, the lesson could be learnt. Say an injury had occurred to the spotter, what actions might you reasonably urge on management in order to prevent recurrences?

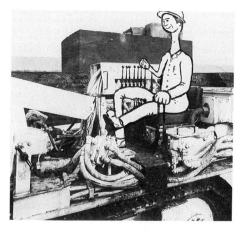

Fig. 5.2   Man designed specifically by ergonomist to operate complex mining machine.
(Courtesy of Mr Steve Mason and Mr Geoff Simpson).

Actions might be divided into immediate and long term. Immediate ones might include clear instructions and education on operation in the presence of a spotter, the use of video equipment instead of a man, and installation of emergency stop buttons. Long-term solutions would involve the provision of ergonomic guidelines for designers, so that future machines could be designed with the needs of the operator in mind. Such guidelines take account of the size, shape and capabilities of workers in relation to the required tasks.

From a medical point of view, the greatest contributions of ergonomics are apparent in the prevention of three very common work-related problems – accidental injury, musculo-skeletal disease, and stress-related illness. When it is realized that these make up the bulk of work-related ill-health, it becomes clear that ergonomics has an important and generally, as yet, underutilized role in preventive workplace medicine.

Case History 5.3

A 45 year-old man was employed as an operative on a production line in a food factory. In a previous period of employment with the company he had spent some time off sick with back pain. Nevertheless, his job entailed collecting waste in plastic buckets from 9, often inaccessible, points in the line. When the line was faulty, as many as 180 buckets needed to be collected on a shift, whereas on a good day as few as 18 were required. When full the buckets weighed 67 kg and were dragged to a main collection point where they were stacked 3 high on a pallette for collection.

In the course of this work, the man (who was of short stature) sustained a prolapsed intervertebral disc. Back and leg pain were still present 2 years after the episode and had prevented his return to work.

This story, with minor variations, is a very frequent one, although methods of prevention rely largely on the application of common sense. We shall return to these later – in the meantime, perhaps you can think out an appropriate strategy for prevention of back injury in physical work. One such is given at the end of the section on ergonomics and prevention (page 114).

Case history 5.4

A 30 year-old lady felt an acute pain in her wrist when propping herself up in bed in the morning. The pain subsided and she went to work in the office of a major insurance company. Her job had involved adding figures and keeping books, but she had recently been transferred to other clerical duties and spent much of the day at a computer keyboard. She had never been shown how to use this in any formal way. After a week she found that the pain in her wrist was getting worse and she had to consult her general practitioner. He certified her sickness absence from work, and prescribed anti-inflammatory drugs and a splint. The pain persisted, perhaps partly because of her need to do housework and look after a young child at home. Referral to an orthopaedic surgeon and a rheumatologist followed, and the term 'repetitive strain syndrome', with its implication of prolonged and even permanent disability, was used. The general practitioner referred her to an occupational physician who examined her and found no physical signs, but an awkward typing technique. He was able to reassure her that she was, by then, recovering from a mild ligamentous strain exacerbated by bad typing techniques. He arranged a rehabilitation programme with the company (including keyboard training) and advised that it review its arrangements for training keyboard operators. Followed up, 2 months after return to work, she was symptom-free.

This story illustrates several common problems in occupational medicine. A mild condition is often made worse by bad work technique or posture. Lack of training and sudden introduction to work with which people are unfamiliar often leads to injury. Multiple medical opinions, especially if uncertain or negative lead to anxiety, which in turn increases perception of symptoms. Positive action and optimism often lead to improvement.

Sometimes, a failure to apply ergonomics can have devastating consequences. Indeed, many of the major disasters that occur in industry can be traced back to a problem in the area of interaction between people and their workplaces.

Case history 5.5

The roll-on, roll-off ferry left the harbour in keeping with its tight timetable. The captain had no warning light on the bridge to tell him whether the bow doors were open or closed, but relied on messages passed by fallible humans. On that night the system failed, the doors were open and the *Herald of Free Enterprise* capsized, drowning 188 people.

In retrospect, it is often the case that the means of preventing such disasters are so obvious that it is hard to understand why they were not employed. Given a design of ship which would allow it to capsize if water entered the hold, it would be thought that automatic, fail-safe mechanisms would have been installed to indicate bow door closure. If, as in this case, consideration of ergonomics at the design stage does not take place, and the necessary measures are not built in, their installation later involves decisions balancing additional costs against likely benefits. Such accidents are, until they occur, often regarded as extremely unlikely and therefore it is easy to come to a decision which prevents excessive expenditure. Clearly this is especially likely in a very competitive situation, where marginal costs must be minimized and therefore risks must increase. The tragic irony in the name of the ship should serve as a reminder of these dangers to all involved in health and safety.

Case history 5.6

In the early hours of the morning in Harrisburg, USA, two operators misread a dial and failed to comprehend the true state of affairs developing at the Three Mile Island nuclear reactor. The problem was accentuated by a number of separate alarms going off simultaneously. Subsequent investigation of this accident, which fortunately caused little damage to health, showed the central problem to have been a failure to ensure that the control panel complied with ergonomic principles, such that under conditions of stress the operators found they were unable to understand and react appropriately to warnings.

A whole area of ergonomics concerns itself with the design of control systems, be they aeroplane cockpits or the control rooms of diving operations or nuclear power stations. It is not uncommon to find such complex arrays of dials and warning signals in the charge of a relatively unsophisticated worker who has not been thoroughly trained, particularly with respect to emergency reactions. Proper design of such systems depends on an understanding of the capabilities and reactions of the operator, and training should involve practice in emergency responses, as in the flight simulators used by airlines.

Ergonomics and prevention

In preventing illness and injury due to work and the workplace, greatest emphasis must be placed on appropriate design of the job, backed by proper education and training of the workers. Selection of appropriate workers is also sometimes necessary, though this is a matter that should only be considered after every attempt has been made to reduce risks in the design of the job.

Job design

Most ergonomic problems in a workplace come to light as a result of sickness absence or complaints by the workers. Almost all are caused by physical or psychological stresses above a threshold acceptable to the workers involved. Many can be traced back to bad, or careless, decisions by managers who had not thought out the implications of these decisions on the workers, and often when the decisions have been implemented it becomes very difficult to resolve the problems. A good example of this has been the 'office revolution', with widespread moves to computers and visual display units.

Case history 5.7

A 50 year-old female records clerk in a hospital was referred to the occupational physician because of prolonged sickness absence. She had been employed for over 20 years with a very good work record, until two years previously. Then, after a series of short absences, she had been off work for 6 months with depression. She had seen a psychiatrist who believed problems at work lay behind her illness. In fact, the source of the problem was the sudden introduction of a computer to make her record keeping more efficient. She was given one day of training and then had to get on with the new job. Having never used a keyboard before she was slow, and felt the younger clerks in the office were laughing at her. Far from making her job easier, the computer added problems to a job which she had previously done without difficulty and contributed largely to her psychological breakdown.

This story had a happy ending, thanks to the ability of a sympathetic manager to adjust her job so as to retain her valuable services. The problem in both these cases arose from a sudden requirement to take on tasks for which the worker had not been adequately trained. These problems do not arise because of an intrinsic design fault of the hardware; rather they are a consequence of its careless introduction and use. After all, secretaries have used typewriters for a century without great problems, and a whole generation of adults has now grown up accustomed to staring at television screens. But the widespread introduction of these devices into workplaces means that many, possibly most, people using keyboards do so without the training that secretaries go through, while the very number of visual display units means that ergonomic factors such as lighting and seating may be quite difficult and costly to bring up to appropriate standards.

The design of a job in such a way as to minimize ergonomic difficulties should include consideration of the factors given in Table 5.1, but always in the light of the capabilities, physical and mental, of the employees. The consequences of not doing so may lead, on the physical side, to musculo-skeletal injury, on the psychological side, to anxiety and depression and on both accounts to increased accident rates.

There is clearly no such thing as an ideal job able to be coped with and enjoyed by all employees, no matter how physically or psychologically vulnerable. Moreover, just as an element of physical work is desirable to

Table 5.1   Some important ergonomic factors in job design

Physical
Loads to be managed weight, dimensions, frequency, etc.
Rate of work
Hours of work and overtime, shift pattern
Breaks, days off and holidays
Postures and range of movements required
Temperature, lighting, noise and vibration
Ventilation

Psychological
Relations with managers and supervisors
Relations with fellow workers
Demands to produce – piece work, bonuses, etc.
Demands upon intellect
Demands when breakdown or emergencies occur
Lack of demand, or boring repetitive work

---

maintain health, so an element of psychological challenge is necessary to promote interest and enthusiasm and to ensure maximum productivity. On the physical side, information is often available which can allow managers to decide what can and cannot sensibly be done by workers. Much of this comes from the science of anthropometry.

Anthropometry deals with measurement of body size and movement. Its importance in ergonomics relates to its role in ensuring appropriate design of tasks and machines. It is, for example, possible from a survey of a workforce to define the range of height, reach in various directions and strength of selected muscle groups, and thus to ensure that given tasks or operations within given workplaces are within the capabilities of actual and potential workers. Such surveys are conventionally described in terms of the capabilities or characteristics of the 5th to 95th percentiles, or 90 per cent of the population, and may apply to any aspect of human physique and performance. Static anthropometry leads to the production of limiting values for dimensions, say, of furniture, equipment and buildings. A familiar use is in the design of car seats and controls. Dynamic anthropometry considers functional operation, and includes posture, range of movement, strength, endurance, precision and sight lines, as well as assessment of capabilities in a psychological sense. It is particularly important in the design of tasks, such as keyboard operation, as well as of controls, such as the keyboard itself.

Case history 5.8

A 25 year-old man presented for a pre-employment medical examination prior to enrolling in a nursing degree course. His previous employment had been in the drilling team on an oil rig. He was a fit looking, muscular man, but had to be turned down on the basis of recurrent back injury which made him physically unsuitable for nurse training.

The injury had occurred on the oil rig, an environment notable for the machismo of some of its workers. He had been told to haul 70 kg segments of metal piping a height of some 10 metres. This he did with a rope, which his mate tied round the objects while he leant over and pulled them up. While doing this he developed acute lumbar pain and sciatica. After a period off work he returned to the job and again injured his back doing another lifting task. Apparently, no consideration had been given to the use of pulleys to lighten a task which required considerable force in an anatomically inefficient posture.

In such cases, the need for lifting aids is often intuitively obvious. For managers and doctors reponsible for workers involved in physical tasks, however, there are published ergonomic guidelines and criteria which can be applied allowing minimization of risk.

Case history 5.9

Back injuries are the most frequent cause of long-term sickness absence in the mining industry. Contrary to popular conceptions, much of the activity underground relates to transport and the operation of complex machinery. As part of a systematic investigation of the ergonomics of underground transport, ergonomists found that cabs in some locomotives were designed with no thought to the dimensions or capabilities of the operators. Controls were badly sited (Fig 5.3), access was difficult; and seats in the cab tended to be a pad of plastic material set on a metal ledge. The postures adopted in operating these machines were such as to suggest a high risk of back injury.

Anthropometric surveys of working miners allowed definition of the appropriate size of the cab, its furniture, controls and doorway. Subsequent redesign of new cabs, using this information, led to a much improved environment for the driver and also gave a potential commercial advantage to the manufacturer.

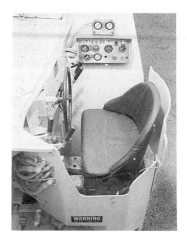

Fig. 5.3   A badly designed workspace in an underground haulage machine

In carrying out such surveys, it is important to take account of factors such as clothing or protective equipment, which may limit reach and mobility, and the requirements of the task itself, which may require a particular type of person. For example, there is little point in trying to redesign the tasks in a rugby scrum so that front row can be anything other than 100 kg mesomorphs – sometimes the task dictates the type of person required. However, in most cases in industry this does not apply, as efficient tools and good design of workplaces allow most tasks to be carried out by people of most shapes and sizes.

In some workplaces, problems are remarkably common. It is interesting that as work in the developed world has shifted from heavy physical activity into the office, so the complaints of work-related ill-health come increasingly from the latter source. The design of office work affords a good example of the application of ergonomics, as outlined in Table 5.1.

The office environment is based increasingly on electronic systems. While these have brought great efficiencies and benefits (who would now go back to re-typing draft after draft of papers?), they have also brought problems. Some are outlined in Table 5.2, analogous to the factors described in Table 5.1.

Such problems tend to become focused in particular workplaces on one factor – for example, the visual display unit or the ventilation systems – and sometimes acquire notoriety as 'sick building syndrome'. Most can be prevented with a little forethought. There are now well established guidelines on the introduction and use of office technology, based on ergonomic criteria. For example, the layout of screen, separate keyboard, document holder and chair should provide maximum flexibility so that the user can adapt them to personal requirements. The chair should be adjustable, stable but mobile, and usually have arm rests. The screen should be positioned so that it does not reflect light. Work should be arranged so that long continuous periods of keyboard operation are avoided, breaks being agreed during which other tasks (such as filing) are performed.

The psychological problems are less easy to prevent, depending largely on skilled management. One very important factor is consultation between managers and operatives before new systems are introduced, followed by a run-in period during which problems are dealt with and workers are given proper training. Only in these circumstances will the full benefits be realized and antagonism be avoided. It is extraordinary how often the authors have encountered intractible workplace problems stemming from neglect of this simple procedure, which sometimes stems from managers' own unfamiliarity with, and even fear of, new technology.

A strategy for prevention of biomechanical injury

On page 108 it was suggested that you might outline a strategy for prevention of back injury at work. This should consider design of the job, so as to minimize awkward postures or loads, training of the workers in safe

Table 5.2   Ergonomic problems in the modern office environment

---

Physical
Frequent repetitive movements at keyboard
High throughput of documents
Awkward postures at desk
Reflection from VDU screen, poor image contrast
Flicker from lights
Background noise
Unsatisfactory temperature and humidity control
Other people's smoke

Psychological
Demanding or unsympathetic managers
Rivalries and animosities between workers
Fear of new technology
Lack of career prospects

---

handling techniques, supervision or audit to ensure that the lessons learnt in training are applied, and selection of appropriate workers, giving special attention to previous history of back injury. In Britain, new Manual Handling Operations Regulations require employers to make an assessment of likely risks involved in operations involving handling loads and to take steps to minimize those risks by redesign of the job, providing appropriate lifting aids and so on.

Ergonomics and illness management

While the primary role of ergonomics is in the prevention of work-related illness and accidents, it also has an important role in management of such conditions. Wherever ergonomic factors have played a part in causing symptoms, or run the risk of exacerbating them, alleviation is usually only possible if the job is redesigned or if the patient spends time off work, perhaps permanently. Again, musculo-skeletal and psychological diseases contribute the bulk of problems where job improvement is necessary.

Job improvement

Work may give rise to either acute or chronic musculo-skeletal disorders. The acute damage is usually, though not necessarily correctly, attributed to an isolated incident of load handling, e.g., lifting a heavy load. The more chronic pattern of presentation arises from repetitive work/movements, sometimes known by the American term 'cumulative damage'. Often, however, the acute disorder is in fact the end stage of a degenerative/cumulative process and so the two types tend to merge in practice.

The main sites of pain resulting from awkward postures or movements are the cervical and lumbar spine, the shoulders, elbows and wrists. Problems with the hips and other lower limb joints are much less common, though long-term degenerative disease of these joints may well be contributed to by physical activity at work. The interrelations between such activity and trauma are complex, since a reasonable level of activity is likely to be protective by ensuring good muscularity and, in early adult life, bone development. In women such activity probably also contributes to lessening risks of post-menopausal osteoporosis. The brunt of repetitive trauma seems to fall on the arms and spine, and is generally related to use of excessive force often in an inefficient anatomical position. Again, what is excessive and what is inefficient are matters that may be defined by ergonomics.

Orthopaedic surgeons see a range of conditions affecting the musculo-skeletal system, often apparently of mysterious aetiology. The workplace is one, though far from the only, cause of many of these syndromes. The general practitioner and the occupational physician tend to see conditions at an earlier stage in their development, when their effects and severity are insufficient to fit them into a clear diagnostic category. At this stage, the application of sensible ergonomic principles may often prevent serious injury or chronic disease.

Case history 5.10

A 55 year-old worker in a citric acid factory was employed in a process drying calcium citrate in a centrifuge. The material was caked to the sides of the tub of the centrifuge, and he had to break it up prior to shovelling it out. He consulted his general practitioner because of a painful right hand which was impairing his ability to work, and was diagnosed as having trigger finger. The factory nurse suspected this might be related to his job, and asked the occupational physician to investigate. The patient had tenderness and crepitation over the palmar flexor tendons of his right hand, and obvious triggering of his right ring and little fingers. When asked to show the physician his job, he demonstrated how he repeatedly drove a chisel into the concretions of chemical, using the palm of his right hand to drive the chisel down. Study of the task clearly indicated the cause – the tools being used were not suited to the task, and a powered chisel was introduced. The worker was transferred temporarily to non-manual work and over the next three months his symptoms and signs gradually and completely disappeared.

Had such a patient been referred to a surgeon, who may have believed from reading the literature that work does not cause trigger finger, the outcome might have been less satisfactory and others might have gone on to get the same condition. Many such syndromes may be seen in the workplace and their solution found by an ergonomic assessment. These pains may assume considerable significance to workers as a consequence of anxiety about possible long-term consequences, particularly when there is media publicity about such syndromes as 'tenosynovitis' and 'repetitive strain syndrome'.

As in the above example, the doctor becomes aware of an ergonomic problem when a patient presents with a complaint of ill-health. If the connection between job and illness is made, cure will depend on appropriate modification of the task. Consider the following case history:

Case history 5.11

Two ladies, one aged 20 and the other 46 consulted their general practitioners. The younger had shoulder and neck pains, the older an acute attack of sciatica provoked by lifting a bicycle out of her car boot. Both were treated symptomatically and returned to their work in the hospital central sterilizing department. Their symptoms continued and they contacted their union representative, believing that their work was contributing to their problems.

The occupational physician was asked to see the two patients. He found no abnormal signs in the younger, while the older had some paraspinal muscle spasm and limited flexion, with a reduced straight leg raising test on the right. Both attributed their current symptoms to the use of a new washing machine in the department.

At this stage, what do you think is the appropriate action? What would you do if you were the doctor?

A detailed history revealed that the machine had been in place for about a month, and the workers were finding some difficulties in using it. One said that it was slower than the previous method, which had involved washing the theatre equipment by hand at a bench.

Clearly, a workplace visit was necessary. The physician asked what was the busiest time, and made the visit then – at 8 am the next day. He found that the machine had been introduced without attention to the size and strengths of the workers. Trays had to be lifted from the floor onto the belt of the machine, loaded at a height which was barely possible for the smaller workers, then unloaded at the far end in a mechanically inefficient position. The tray was then lifted off and carried to a trolley. The positions adopted were easily seen to put unnecessary strain on the back and shoulders (Fig. 5.4).

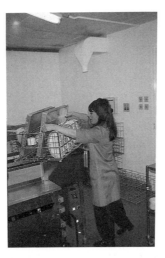

Fig. 5.4 Bad ergonomics. A short operator in a hospital sterilising department having to fill and empty trays on a washing machine at the extreme limit of her reach

The machine was a big investment and was fixed. What could be done? In fact, the solutions were quite simple.

The physician noted that the heights of the workers, all female, ranged from 4ft 8ins to 5ft 6ins. The job rotation pattern required all to take a 2-week turn on the machine, loading for one week and unloading for another week, every 6 weeks. He suggested that trays were stacked on a table at the loading end, so no bending and twisting was required, the trays simply being carried across at chest height. A platform was recommended at the unloading end for the shorter workers, and the trays were orientated so that articles were pulled out towards, rather than away from, the woman on unloading duties. Finally, the trolley was placed adjacent to the belt at the unloading end, so that trays could simply be lifted across rather than carried.

Such common sense management hardly justifies the title ergonomics, but the benefits are potentially great. In this situation, one worker was at serious risk of recurrence of her sciatica (incidentally, she was transferred to lighter duties temporarily) and others were likely to develop intractible muscular discomfort which would eventually lead to sickness absence, resignations and possibly litigation. All could have been prevented by application of ergonomics in the design of the job and the machine. It appeared, rather typically, that it had been designed by men for men!

Another point is raised by this story. The older patient went back to her work rather too early, prompted by the need to maximise her income. If you had been her general practitioner, and had some concerns about her ability to cope with a physical task, you would have had three options: to send her back and hope for the best, to advise her not to go back, or to contact her manager about a rehabilitation period. This last important, but rarely considered, option is discussed fully in Chapter 8. If, as in this case, the organization has an occupational physician, the patient could have been referred for an opinion.

Occupational hygiene

The discipline of occupational hygiene is concerned with the recognition, evaluation and control of hazard in the working environment. Its practitioners usually come from a background of chemistry, engineering or physics, although biologists and nurses are increasingly being attracted to the discipline. In some countries, such as those in Eastern Europe, it may be a medical specialty. It is usual in large organizations for an occupational hygienist to work closely with physician, nurse and safety officer towards the common goal of ensuring a safe workplace.

The four essential stages to the practice of occupational hygiene are:

- recognition of hazardous work situations or practices
- measurement of the levels of pollutant or stressor
- design and implementation of control measures
- audit of effectiveness of controls.

Recognition

The methods of approaching and examining a workplace have been outlined in Chapter 3. Each stressor or pollutant in the working environment can be classified into one of several classes.

(a) Physical   These agents include noise and vibration, visible and ultraviolet light, microwaves, ionizing radiation and heat and cold, dependent on incident energy for their effects. In this category of physical hazards one may include the biomechanical stresses, of primary interest to ergonomists, discussed above.

(b) Chemical   The worker may be exposed to inorganic and organic chemicals in a diversity of physical states as dust, fume, gas, vapour and mist. The toxic agent must gain access to the body, usually by inhalation or percutaneously, in order to have a significant health effect. In each occupational setting, the risk to the individual arises as a function of toxicity and the level of exposure, which determines the dose over time. Not only must the toxic agent be present, but it must be absorbed in sufficient quantities to create a toxic effect at the critical organ.

(c) Biological   Biological agents may cause illness in consequence of their infective or toxic nature, or of their capacity to act as antigens and produce a harmful immune response. In recent years biological agents have achieved greater prominence in the workplace, most notably *Legionella sp* in air conditioning systems and the viruses responsible for Hepatitis B and HIV, a source of concern for health care and some public service workers. The importance of animal and plant antigens, especially the former, as sensitizers has been recognized more widely also.

(d) Psychological   Stress in the workplace is responsible for much ill health, as has been discussed in Chapter 2 and in the section on ergonomics.

Evaluation

In Chapter 3 we discussed how to approach a workplace visit. Often the assessment of risk from perceived hazards depends on some form of measurement of the workplace environment. In making such measurements, the hygienist (or ergonomist) will bear in mind the type of hazard and its possible effects on workers. It will also be necessary to know something of the variability of the hazard over time and of any measures taken to protect workers. What ultimately is important is the dose of hazard which the individual takes up, and which is determined by exposure. However, individual susceptibility to a given dose may vary considerably.

Sampling

In order to evaluate risk, the first requirement is to obtain representative measurements in relation to the activities of workers. This is not possible without a detailed knowledge of the whole of the task performed by individuals – not infrequently an otherwise apparently safe process becomes unsafe as a consequence of a seemingly trivial procedure.

Case history 5.12

A young man presented to his doctor with a history of nervousness, frequency of micturition and trembling. He had associated this with his work, which involved testing samples of oil for gas content. The process was enclosed and took place under mercury, which he injected from a container. Great care was taken to monitor air levels of mercury in the workplace and blood and urine samples from the workers were also being monitored regularly. His had shown a steady and unexplained rise.

On detailed review of his work, it transpired that at the end of each analytical procedure it was necessary to flush any residual gas out of the enclosed system. This was done in such a way that any residual mercury could have volatilized and been discharged into the air of the workplace. Indeed such transient peaks were apparent on close inspection of the monitoring records. Subsequent control of this part of the process alleviated the problem.

This case history illustrates that a meticulous approach to assessing working practices is essential to good preventive occupational medicine. Even regular monitoring may be insufficient if inadequate attention is paid to its siting, timing or, as in this case, the results.

Measurement of environmental hazards ideally might be made continuously, on-line, from multiple fixed points where the hazard is estimated to be most likely to be present. Such systems were widely introduced for the measurement of vinyl chloride monomer in PVC plants after the risk of hepatic angiosarcoma was recognized. Levels above those allowed would then trigger an alarm and allow prompt action to be taken. Similar systems are in use, for example, for gases in mining and the petrochemical industries. At the other extreme of sampling strategy, one may use a wide array of portable equipment to measure gases, noise, radiation and so on. A number of the commonly used pieces of apparatus are illustrated (Fig. 5.5).

Since it is the dose of the hazard that reaches the worker that is important, personal sampling devices are available for a wide range of chemical substances and physical hazards. The most familiar to a doctor is the radiation badge (or personal dosimeter), which measures cumulative exposure to ionizing radiation. Personal noise meters are also available. Gas and dust samplers are usually operated by a pump, attached to the belt, sucking air through a tube of absorbent granules or a filter device on the worker's lapel. Methods for assessing skin exposure to chemicals are so far not available, however.

Standards

The act of sampling workplace air of course implies that the measurements

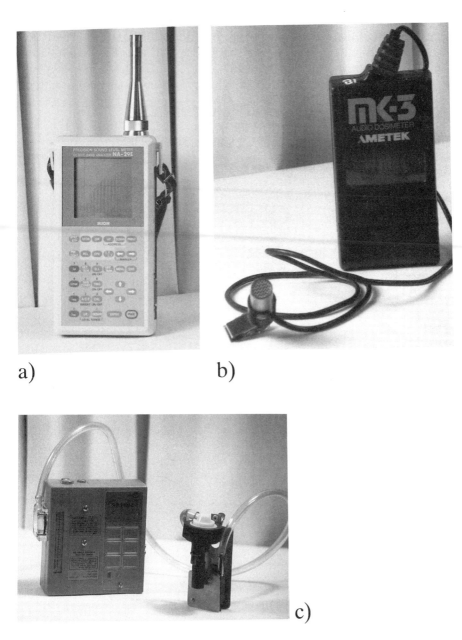

a)

b)

c)

Fig. 5.5 (a) Sound level meter with octave band analyser. Used to measure the sound level and frequency spectrum at a fixed location. (b) Personal sound dosemeter which is used to measure average sound level for an individual worker. The microphone can be clipped close to the ear and the electronic unit attached to the wearer's belt. (c) Personal sampling pump and sampling head for respirable dust. The pump can be clipped to the wearer's belt and the sampling head attached to the lapel, close to the nose and mouth. The dust is collected inside the sampling head on a filter paper.

obtained mean something in terms of threats to health, in the same way as measurement of blood constituents indicates disease in a patient. There thus needs to be some guidance on the harmfulness of specific levels of toxic substances. While it could be argued that the only safe level of, say, mercury, is no mercury, such guidance lacks practicality in many workplace situations.

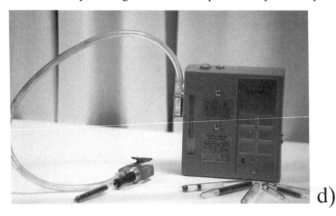

d)

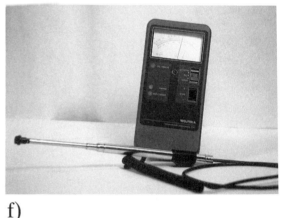

f)

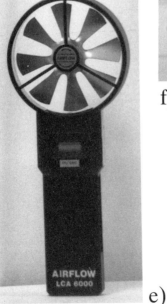

e)

Fig. 5.5 *(cont.)* (d) Personal sampling pump and sampling head for gases and vapours. The pump unit is the same as for dusts, although operated at a lower flow rate. The sampling head consists of a glass tube containing an adsorbent, specific to the gas or vapour being sampled. A selection of adsorbent tubes is also shown. (e) Vane anemometer used to measure average air velocity at the entrance to fume cupboards and other ventilation systems. (f) Hot wire anemometer used to measure air velocity in ventilation ducts and other moving air streams.

A small number of carcinogenic substances are regarded as too toxic to handle, and are therefore banned, but most other harmful substances are believed safe enough to use if levels are kept below a stated maximum. The concept that there is for such substances a threshold, below which harm is unlikely to occur, gave rise to the term *'threshold limit value'* (TLV) which is still used in

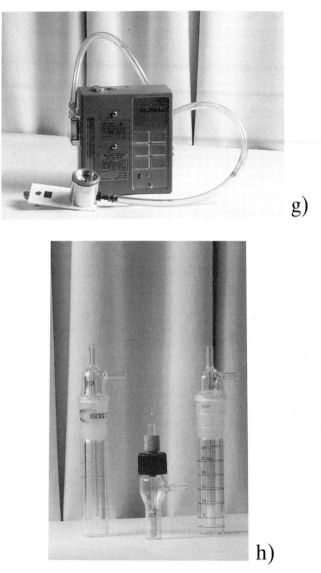

g)

h)

Fig. 5.5 *(cont.)* (g) Personal sampling pump and sampling head for lead dust. The pump can be clipped to the wearer's belt and the sampling head attached to the lapel, close to the nose and mouth. The dust is collected inside the sampling head on a filter paper. (h) Glass impingers and bubblers, used with a pump to collect gases or vapours and some particulates. The glass tubes are filled with an appropriate absorbing solution and air is then passed through the liquid. (Photographs courtesy of Mr John Cherrie).

the USA. Two sorts of TLV are published in that country for a wide range of airborne substances – one which gives a figure averaged over an 8-hour period, and a short-term (or ceiling) value which should not be exceeded over a short period.

In Britain, standards are published by the Health and Safety Executive, and are called '*occupational exposure limits*' (OELs). These come in two lists, '*maximal exposure limits*' (MELs), which includes substances of known serious toxicity and sets standards which must not be exceeded, and '*occupational exposure standards*' (OES), which gives levels at which there is no evidence of harm to workers exposed over a working lifetime. The OES list includes many substances of lesser toxicity. It is important to recognize that the MEL does not guarantee safety – it may well be set at a level at which there is still a finite risk to health.

Standards of whatever type vary from country to country, and from time to time within a country. They are based upon a combination of epidemiological and experimental evidence as far as possible, but ultimately are often arrived at through discussion, speculation and consideration of safety factors in the absence of any human toxicology. Moreover, economic factors, namely the extent to which industry or society can afford to comply, often influence the setting of an exposure limit. They should therefore be looked upon as guidance for control measures rather than as absolute 'safe levels', and steps should always be taken to keep actual levels as far below such standards as practicable. Examples of some current UK standards are given in Appendix 2.

Control

When asked to discuss methods of preventing occupational disease, most doctors and students instinctively start by mentioning methods of personal protection, such as ear muffs or respirators.

Think for a moment why this is the wrong approach. Say, for example, a farmer had told you to use an arsenic-containing chemical to kill the parasites on his flock of sheep during a summer job as a student, what measures might you sensibly have taken to protect yourself? Personal protection has several disadvantages – it is never 100 per cent efficient (and rarely even 50 per cent), it depends on the full cooperation of the wearer, it requires careful maintenance, it may interfere with the task, and it may induce complacency. Better surely, in our example, not to use arsenic. Substitution of safer for less safe substances is the first step to consider. Other steps may include enclosure of processes and exhaust and dilution ventilation.

Case history 5.13

The sister in a gastroenterology unit became unable to enter the endoscopy suite, for which she was responsible, because of rhinitis, lacrimation and wheeze. She reported that she had had to delegate cleaning of the endoscopes to a staff nurse who developed similar symptoms. Others in the unit complained of sore eyes. The cause was glutaraldehyde (which is currently considered necessary to prevent possible transmission of Hepatitis B and HIV), used in an open container and syringed down the endoscopes. The occupational physician watched the whole procedure, which involved at one stage holding the endoscopes up at arm's length, the glutaraldehyde running down the arm of the nurse. He advised on the provision of an exhaust ventilation cabinet, equipped with appropriate sinks. The doctors on the unit preferred to purchase a special machine for washing the endoscopes – this did the job more efficiently but did not eliminate the source of exposure, and ultimately exhaust ventilation was installed over the machine itself.

This story illustrates the fact that the obvious solution is not always the best one. Prior to the request for advice from the occupational physician, the unit staff had decided that better ventilation was the answer, and had the hospital engineer instal an extractor fan. Unfortunately this was put in the ceiling, about 3 metres above the source of vapour, and simply drew air from the door 6 metres away to the ceiling, leaving the vapour to eddy round the nurse's face. Then the consultants thought that if the process were automated, exposure would cease. This did not take account of the facts that the machine had to be filled and emptied and that vapour of glutaraldehyde was able to escape from it. To avoid contact between people and vapour, it was necessary for the vapour to be drawn away from the person, and an extractor cabinet was an effective way of doing this. One final problem occurred in this extraordinary episode – an ergonomic one. In spite of advice on design, the engineers built a cabinet with the sink so far to the rear that the nurses, who were of short stature, had to put their upper body inside to reach it (Fig. 5.6)! Fortunately this was spotted before the unit was used and was able to be corrected.

The principles of control of exposure to harmful substances are therefore:

1. **Substitution** of a less harmful for a more harmful substance or operation. Important examples in industry have been the substitution of toluene or cyclohexane for benzene, chalk for talc and mineral wools for asbestos.

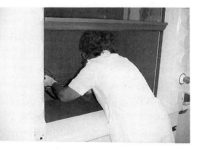

Fig. 5.6 Fume cupboard in endoscopy unit – designed so that nurses have to put their heads inside in order to wash endoscopes!

Where the harm comes from a contaminant or a by-product, for example benzidine in organic dyes, it may be possible to specify a maximum content of the contaminant. Noise injury may also be prevented by specification in the design of new machinery.

2. **Segregation** of workers from the source of harm. This may be by time or distance, as in mining where workers retire to a safe distance at the time of blasting, and when such operations take place on shifts when fewer workers are about. More commonly, however, it involves enclosure of the process so that there is a physical barrier between the source of harm and the workers.

3. **Local exhaust ventilation** is used where the above methods are impracticable. Ideally it is combined with partial enclosure of the process, as in the familiar fume cabinet. Alternatively, the ventilation is applied very close to the point of generation of the dust or vapour. The air velocity required to draw the substance away is called the capture velocity, and this depends on the physical characteristics of the substance and the mechanisms of its release. It is intuitively obvious that lower velocities are needed to clear evaporating chemicals than particles generated by blasting or drilling.

4. Reduction of airborne levels of substances by **dilution ventilation or precipitation**. A familiar example is the use of water and high air flows in mines to reduce dust levels. Electrostatic forces may also be used to reduce levels of dust, commonly in preventing pollution by smoke stacks.

5. **Personal protection.** The law generally requires all reasonable efforts be made to engineer the hazard out or to shield individuals from it. Only then is it permissible to resort to personal protection. Most such devices are not comfortable for long-term use and give only partial protection. Included in this category are respirators, protective clothing and gloves, eye shields and hearing defenders. Clearly in some circumstances they are mandatory – eye protection in welding and metal work, ear muffs in caulking (which today means hammering metal in ships' hulls), and so on. However, they should never be relied upon as the sole, albeit cheap, method of protecting workers. Where they are used, care should be taken in their design, in terms of comfort and wearability, as well as in their efficiency in terms of protection. Some forms of personal protection and their efficiencies are illustrated (Fig. 5.7).

6. **Education and good housekeeping** remain important principles of prevention in all circumstances. Workers should be made aware of dangers by instruction, notices, codes of practice and safety audit. Similarly, managers should be trained in their responsibilities in these respects. Good housekeeping, keeping chemicals in safe places, not leaving dangerous materials (or indeed any materials) lying about, making sure that everything is clearly labelled, vacuuming floors and benches after use, and other such measures will reduce risks of illness and accident and will ensure that everyone is safety-conscious.

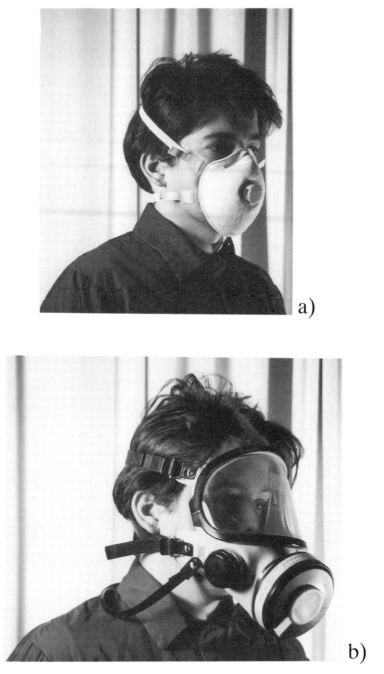

Fig. 5.7   (a) Filtering facepiece respirator to provide a moderate level of protection against dusts and other aerosols. (b) Full face powered respirator which will provide a high degree of protection against dusts and other aerosols.

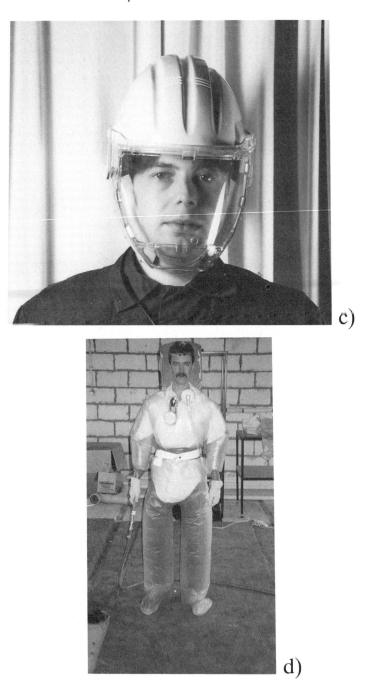

(c) Powered helmet respirator. Air is drawn from behind the head, filtered to remove any particles and blown over the face. The unit also provides head protection and a visor to protect the
face. (d) Ventilated suit used to provide higher level of respiratory and body protection against
radioactive dust. (Photographs courtesy of Mr John Cherrie).

Problems with control measures

None of these methods is flawless and several should normally be used in combination. Can you think of problems with each of them? Some real life examples may surprise you.

Substitution The widespread substitution of solvents such as toluene and white spirit for the leukaemogenic benzene has given rise to the concept of 'safe' solvents. However these substances are only relatively safe, and their uncontrolled use may lead to neurological or psychological disease, as described in Chapter 2. Similarly, certain fibrous minerals used as substitutes for asbestos may themselves have carcinogenic potential, and require careful handling.

Segregation A case has already been quoted (Chapter 1, history 1.5) in which an organic dye process was properly enclosed, but fitters required access for maintenance and repair. One of these men subsequently developed bladder cancer. Similarly, in a very clean and well-kept bakery the only man who developed asthma due to flour allergy was the fitter who had to repair pipes and silos when they burst. Remember, when looking at a well isolated piece of machinery, to ask how it is maintained or repaired.

Exhaust ventilation This is very effective if properly designed and if the extractor fan is working. A young female technician developed allergic alveolitis and asthma due to sensitization to a chemical reagent she was preparing in a fume cupboard in the laboratory of a university medical school. When the problem was investigated, it was found the extractor fan was not working. Three men developed acute mercury poisoning while making repairs in the boiler of a power station. Some other workers in a distant part of the plant had spilt some mercury which had vaporized. The extract fan in the system was running in reverse and the vapour was propelled along pipes to the boiler in which the other men were working.

Dilution Here the substance remains in the air, but in lower concentration. Unforseen problems may however occur to make matters worse. An operating theatre had a well-designed ventilation system to reduce microbial levels in the area around the patient. Nevertheless, a series of patients undergoing prosthetic heart valve surgery developed infections with *Aspergillus fumigatus*. It was eventually discovered that the fungal spores were being removed efficiently from the air by filters which needed to be changed regularly. The technician changing these was not given any special instructions, and simply took them down into the theatre, substituting the new ones. This process released the captured spores in high concentration. In other cases, the supply of conditioned, humidified air to operating theatres has resulted in humidifier fever among theatre staff.

Personal protection   Sometimes personal protection devices may be even worse than implied by their efficiencies. Face masks are not as universal in their fitting to the human face as manufacturers and wearers would hope, and thus often allow leakage. Filters on respirators need changing regularly or their performance deteriorates. Some disposable respirators become ineffective after use because of being crumpled in a pocket or soaked with water. Respirators require to be formally tested to various standards – in doing this, testing laboratories have found filters that release respirable fibres, giving higher counts within the masks than outside! Some helmet type respirators become less efficient if used in moderately windy conditions. Ear plugs may contribute to otitis externa, visors may obscure the welding job and thus not be used properly, gloves may be permeable to chemicals, and so on.

Education and good housekeeping   To be effective, as all doctors know, education has to be a continuing process. After three fatal cases of pneumonia had occurred in a biotechnology factory, all managers were instructed in appropriate preventive measures, and codes of practice were introduced for hazardous operations, of which the most important was water spraying. After an illness-free period of four years, another severe case of pneumonia occurred. The victim, who fortunately survived, was a contract worker who had been using a high pressure hose in a cleaning operation. The manager in charge was new, and had not been informed of his responsibilities in

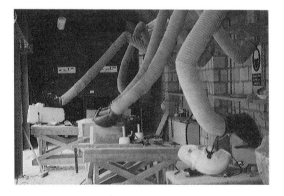

Fig. 5.8 Stonemason's yard – previously seen in Fig. 3.1 – now shown after exhaust ventilation had been installed. The brush propped against a pillar on the right hand side indicates that workers are nevertheless likely to be exposed to high concentrations of dust when sweeping up after masonry work has finished. The helmet respirator has also been carelessly discarded.

supervizing contract workers and preventing such hosing procedures.

Figure 5.8 illustrates a common problem arising from good housekeeping. Can you see what it is?

Immunisation

The need to consider immunisation in an occupational setting arises for three reasons:

- active prevention of a specific, work-related hazard
- passive treatment of a work-related injury
- prophylaxis for overseas travel.

These matters are discussed in detail in Chapters 4 and 9.

The role of worker selection in prevention

While, in general, jobs should be designed so as to make them safe to be carried out by any employee, some of them of necessity involve tasks which are beyond the capabilities of some individuals. Such circumstances lead to the requirement for pre-employment selection procedures. When this is necessary, it is appropriate to think first of the precise physical and psychological demands of the job, and then to decide on appropriate requirements. A familiar example is the selection of medical students. What are the demands placed on a doctor? How far did the selection procedures of your medical school go towards picking out those most capable of doing the job? In retrospect, looking at your experience and that of your fellow students, do you think these procedures could have been more effective?

In many cases in recent years, selection into medical school has been on the basis of results in school examinations alone. This provides a test of intelligence and ability to recall facts, two factors which are undoubtedly important in the practice of medicine, and which probably ensure that a majority of those selected will survive the pre-clinical course. But how far does it select those capable of coping with the stressful early years of training and able to deal effectively with the many years ahead in clinical practice? A moment's thought will allow you to see two possible approaches to this problem – more careful selection, by aptitude and psychological testing, or modification of the tasks. At present in medicine in Britain the emphasis is, probably rightly, on the latter, at least with respect to the many years spent training, where progress has been substantial if rather slow. The former approach has not been seriously considered, and provides interesting research opportunities for the deans of medical schools.

Similar considerations apply in many other jobs, and most include some selection procedures, usually aimed at selecting people who can work most efficiently and effectively. As automation has spread through industry, the emphasis has increasingly turned from physical to mental capabilities, but some jobs still require high standards of physical fitness and it is appropriate to have specific criteria for such work. For example, police and fire fighters, the military and divers all have jobs which may place high physical demands on the individual, and it is appropriate that candidates should measure up to certain defined criteria since it is unlikely that the jobs can ever be made significantly less stressful; physical breakdown of an individual in such jobs could put others at risk.

The essential point is to think first of the criteria for performance and safety relevant to the job, and then to decide on appropriate selection procedures. Regrettably, this is often not the way the matter is approached.

Case history 5.14

A Health Board in the National Health Service decided that its occupational health service should generate income. It had recently decided that it could obtain a more cost-effective hospital cleaning service by contracting it out to a privately owned firm, and decided to write into the contract that all cleaners should have a pre-employment medical examination, for which the company was charged.

The job of hospital cleaner was very poorly paid and often part-time. It therefore attracted people who were only likely to stay until something better turned up. Moreover the work was arduous, as the company had contracted to do the work with fewer people at lower salaries than was previously considered desirable. The consequence was a very high rate of staff turnover. This initially had the effect of producing income for the occupational health service (even if at a considerable waste of nursing and medical time), but did not have any impact on selecting appropriate people for the job. Moreover, after a short period the company realised that it was wasting money on having people examined who would shortly leave their employ, and adopted a tactic of taking workers on first, subsequently referring them for health screening. This ensured that only those likely to stay a reasonable period were examined, and from the company's point of view was a sensible solution, though it caused problems when people were detected to have disease (usually chronic skin conditions) that made them unsuitable for such work.

What went wrong here? The decision to require health screening was made by a manager simply to obtain income, without real thought as to the medical justifications for it. A moment's thought about the medical requirements for hospital cleaning jobs would have led to the conclusion that if anything was needed it would be a written statement from prospective employees that they did not suffer from any of a short list of illnesses, examination being offered only to those who admitted to having one. As it was, a lot of time was wasted to no obvious effect, and the real costs outweighed the value of the income generated.

If you are asked to carry out pre-employment examinations, ask the following questions:

- What are the physical and mental criteria for the job?
- What detectable medical conditions would preclude individuals from that work?
- What is the most cost-effective means of detecting those conditions?

The third question must take account of the likely frequency of the condition in the population, as well as its detectability on physical examination. Most conditions are best detected by a screening questionnaire rather than by medical examination, saving the latter for those who answer positively.

Indiscriminate use of medical screening, usually to generate income, has contributed largely to the low esteem in which occupational medicine has been held by members of other medical specialties. It is important for those practising occupational medicine to consider critically its value in terms of preventing ill-health, mental and physical, before becoming involved in it. Even where a particular constitutional factor has been shown to increase the risk of developing an occupational disease as a result of a given exposure it does not necessarily follow that exclusion from employment on the basis of that factor is justified. Consider the following example:

Substance X can cause occupational asthma, and atopics have twice as high a risk of developing occupational asthma from occupational exposure to it under the prevailing conditions than non-atopics. At your hospital you have a test which will clearly identify a proportion of the applicants as atopics. Thus we have the following contingency table:

	Applicants	*Will develop asthma*	*Will not develop asthma*
'Atopic' by your test	30	6	24
'Non-atopic'	70	7	63
Total	100	13	67

As the above table clearly shows, non-atopics have a 10 per cent chance of developing asthma while for atopics it is 20 per cent.

If you stopped the atopics from being employed:

- How many cases of asthma would you prevent?
- How many cases of asthma would still occur?
- How many people who would not have developed asthma would have been deprived of the opportunity to do that job?
- What could you advise management to do instead of barring atopics from employment?

The law generally requires exposure to be controlled so that 'almost all' the population could be employed day in, day out without an adverse effect on health resulting. Is 70/100 'almost all' the population?

In these circumstances you would probably wish to persuade management to control exposures, by the measures discussed earlier in this chapter, rather than to exclude atopic individuals.

Legislation and prevention of occupational disease

The preventive measures discussed so far rely for their effectiveness on knowledge of risk and a willingness to take action to reduce it. This alone is insufficient, unless it is covered by legal sanctions in the event of negligence leading to injury or illness. Thus, most countries have a framework of health and safety law, backed by a system of enforcement, and analogous to those parts of the criminal law seeking to protect citizens from other forms of violence. In addition, people injured as a result of their work generally have the right to sue their employers in the civil courts for negligently causing such injury, the onus being on the injured party to prove negligence.

Almost all countries have their own legislation, within often widely differing court systems. In this section we discuss the British system, which because of the careful thought that has gone into its more recent framing might be regarded as a model for such legislation and for methods of enforcement. We also refer to systems in the European Community, whose laws take priority over those of the member states, and in the United States of America.

The Health and Safety at Work, etc., Act, 1974

Prior to 1970, British health and safety law was a mess, with some 500 separate pieces of legislation covering a multitude of dangerous substances and situations at work, and administered by nine separate Government departments. It was gradually realized that rigid enforcement of the law would be impracticable, leading to reduction of industrial competitiveness and overload of the court system. The mass of legislation was therefore reviewed by the Robens Committee, which concluded that in spite of this law, there had been no significant reduction in the numbers of people killed and injured at work. A new Act was therefore framed, intended to cover all eventualities by putting a general obligation on employers to ensure, as far as reasonably practicable, the health and safety of their employees. This Act is known as the Health and Safety at Work, etc., Act and the primary responsibility for its enforcement falls on a Cabinet Minister, the Secretary of State for Employment.

Some basic knowledge of the Act is important to all doctors in Britain, since (with the associated Regulations, as discussed later) it embraces all the structures necessary for ensuring the prevention of occupational disease and injury.

The essential features of relevance to doctors are as follows:

- It requires all employers to provide, as far as is reasonably practicable, a healthy and safe workplace.
- It requires employers to take care not only of their employees but also of other people visiting the worksite. This of course includes contractors as well as visitors and paying customers.
- It requires site operators to prevent, as far as practicable, emission of toxic substances into the general atmosphere.
- It requires manufacturers to ensure that their products are reasonably safe, and to provide information on safety precautions to be taken in their use.
- It requires *employees* to take reasonable precautions for the safety of themselves and of others.
- It makes provision for the appointment of trade union or employee safety representatives and requires employers, if requested by such representatives, to set up safety committees.
- It established the Health and Safety Commission (HSC), with a Chairman appointed by the Secretary of State and members appointed after discussion with representatives of industrial management, employees and local Government. The HSC is responsible for administration of the Act, for promoting research, for providing an information and advisory service, and for submitting proposals for Regulations to the Secretary of State.
- It established the executive arm of the HSC, the Health and Safety Executive (HSE), managed by a director and two other members, assisted by area directors. This has responsibility for enforcing the law, having taken over the various original Inspectorates. These include the factories, chemicals, agriculture, offshore oil and gas, nuclear and railways inspectorates, and what used to be the medical branch of the Factories Inspectorate, the Employment Medical Advisory Service (EMAS). EMAS, which includes doctors and nurses trained in occupational medicine, has responsibility for advising the Inspectorates on medical matters, carrying out medical investigation and surveys of workplaces, giving advice to employers and others on occupational medical matters and carrying out research. These EMAS doctors are the specialists to whom British doctors should normally turn for advice when confronted with suspected occupational disease.

Regulations under the Act

There remain a number of Regulations specific to certain particularly dangerous substances, including lead and asbestos, situations, such as underground mining, or physical dangers such as noise and ionizing radiation. Any doctor involved with an organisation or industry in which these hazards arise must be familiar with the relevant Regulations, which give specific guidance on control, monitoring and so on. Otherwise the law has been much simplified by the introduction of the general *Control of Substances Hazardous to Health Regulations, 1988*, widely known by the acronym COSHH. These cover all substances (other than those few, notably lead and asbestos, covered by specific Regulations) with the potential to cause harm in the workplace. The workplace is anywhere where a person might work, and substances include micro-organisms. The Regulations may be summarized quite simply:

- They require an audit of the workplace to detect any potentially harmful substances in use.
- The employer or a representative should then review the use of that substance and decide on whether its use may constitute a significant risk to individuals. If not, a note is simply made of the assessment.
- If a risk appears possible, appropriate steps to reduce the risk should be taken, and a note of these should be made. Regular review of compliance with these procedures is necessary.
- In such circumstances, the employer must consider whether environmental monitoring or surveillance of the workforce is necessary. If either is, again records must be made and kept for up to 40 years.

In general, the emphasis is on control of substances at source, so that workplace monitoring is only required infrequently and worker surveillance very rarely. The latter needs to be considered when there is a reasonable likelihood, in spite of the precautions taken, that workers will develop harmful effects, and that there are valid techniques for detecting the condition when it does occur.

Case history 5.15

Owing presumably to successful promotion by the manufacturers, the use of glutaraldehyde has become widespread in hospitals, and in one such it was found to be used in some 40 different units. It was pointed out to users that they required to make a COSHH assessment in each case, and that this would clearly involve consideration of the use of safer alternatives. Since its only real application is in the sterilization of instruments, such as endoscopes, that could have been contaminated with Hepatitis B or HIV infected blood and that require rapid re-use, it was believed that this would result in a sharp drop in its use. A year later, a repeat survey showed that its use was undiminished and that a COSHH assessment had been done only rarely.

Like all the examples given in this book, this is a true story. If you were the occupational physician in this hospital, what would you have done at this stage? Remember, the Inspectors of the HSE could come in at any time, or a person complaining of symptoms could call in EMAS or even take an action in court against the hospital.

The second survey also revealed that an appreciable number of nurses were suffering symptoms attributable to glutaraldehyde exposure. The hospital administration was advised, again, of the potential risks they were taking with their employees, and it was suggested that they strictly controlled the use of glutaraldehyde to areas where there was no satisfactory alternative. The hospital infection control committee was asked to advise on appropriate alternatives. Extraction and enclosure procedures were instituted where glutaraldehyde was used and all employees working in such areas were required to attend for 6-monthly medical surveillance. Central control of glutaraldehyde dispensing through the pharmacy, and the inconvenience of medical surveillance, resulted in a sharp drop in its use.

The type of surveillance of individuals may vary. It may involve as little as the employer keeping a health record of exposed employees or as much as regular monitoring of blood (e.g., mercury workers) or examination by a doctor. In many cases, questioning and examination by an occupational health nurse is what is required, reporting any suspected problems to a doctor.

All the Regulations, including the new Manual Handling Operations Regulations, take roughly the same practical form, namely

- assess risk
- implement controls to reduce those risks
- provide personal protection only when all other appropriate measures have been taken
- if necessary, provide environmental monitoring and/or surveillance of exposed workers.

It can be seen, for example, with respect to noise in the workplace that the objectives would be to control the level by using quieter machinery or by soundproofing the process and, if this were not wholly effective, to provide ear protection to exposed workers. In such noisy workplaces, it would be wise to monitor levels regularly (a requirement under the Noise at Work Regulations with levels over 90dBA) and to provide audiometric screening of the workforce.

Regulations issued by the Health and Safety Commission with the approval of the Secretary of State for Employment are part of the law and their provisions are mandatory, breach being an offence. However, for the purpose of giving practical guidance, the HSC also issues Codes of Practice covering and explaining the Regulations. These are written in relatively simple language, and are obtainable from Her Majesty's Stationery Office bookshops.

Enforcement

Law is of course useless unless it is seen to be enforced – witness the widespread lack of observance of speed limits in Britain. The role of enforcer of safety and health legislation falls to the Inspectorate of the HSE. Inspectors have wide powers to enter workplaces, to inspect them and take samples and to require premises to be sealed off. If necessary they can obtain the help of the police. They are able to issue enforcement notices of improvement requiring matters to be put right within a specified time, or of prohibition of further activity where circumstances are thought to be particularly dangerous. Employers have the right of appeal against these to Industrial Tribunals.

Much of the work of inspectors involves routine inspection of workplaces and education of employers. They may, however, be contacted by workers, trades unions or others concerned about safety and health hazards at work. In cases of serious breaches of the law, inspectors may take employers or site owners to court, where fines or even imprisonment may be imposed. There has been a welcome tendency in Britain recently for the courts to take such offences, often resulting in loss of life, more seriously and to impose severe punishment. Nevertheless, it remains true that the consequence of killing an employee at work is generally less severe than that of killing someone by dangerous driving.

Legislation in other countries

In the United States the Occupational Safety and Health (OSH) Act was enacted in 1970. Like the later British Act, it puts a general obligation on employers to maintain a safe workplace. The responsibility for enforcement rests on the Department of Labor, through the Occupational Safety and Health Administration (OSHA). OSHA sets workplace standards and has emphasised in particular the regulation of carcinogens. Its powers are similar to those of the British HSE, and it also emphasises voluntary efforts to improve health and safety, providing education and consultative services to industry. The OSH Act also created a research arm, the National Institute of Occupational Safety and Health (NIOSH) as part of the Public Health Service of the Department of Health and Human Services. This organisation also produces Criteria Documents, giving the evidence necessary for standard setting, and provides an information and advice service on occupational health problems. The OSH Act does not cover the self-employed nor, as in Britain, does it cover industries, such as underground coalmining, already covered by separate Acts.

The European Community has embarked on a series of Directives in the field of health and safety, all of which when agreed by the Commission become binding on all the member countries. They have proceeded on the basis of individual hazards, setting standards which are then enforced by the appropriate national agencies. Recent ones include Directives on noise, visual display units, the manual handling of loads, carcinogens and biological agents. European Directives are arrived at by consensus between representatives of the national governments and their experts and, once promulgated, give a time limit within which member nations must comply.

Information, education and training

In some obviously hazardous industries, safety training is well established and effective. For example, it plays an important part in the overall job training of coalminers and seamen. Most nurses receive some training in safe lifting techniques, but many auxiliary nurses do not. In many industries and organisations, information on health and safety is not given to workers.

It is clear that a well-informed, safety conscious worker is less likely to suffer work-related injury or illness than an ignorant one, just as a driver who reads and complies with the provisions of the Highway Code is less likely to have an accident. Safety and health training should be a part of every organization's strategy, its level and intensity being dictated by the perceived risk in the workplace. If the risk is no greater than tripping over or having a heart attack at work, then first aid provision and training is all that is necessary, but in most workplaces, as the reader will by now realize, risks are usually somewhat greater. Upper limb disorders in offices, back injuries in manual workers, deafness in noisy places–all these are preventable by appropriate modifications in the workplace but are more likely to be prevented if the workers are informed of risk and of protective measures. It is not sufficient to leave this to the trade union, whose representatives at shop floor level have sometimes been known to be more interested in negotiating 'danger money' than in ameliorating conditions.

The range of methods of information and education is large, and each organization should plan its own strategy. Joint management-worker safety committees are a useful forum for planning such activity, which may include posters, leaflets, lectures and seminars, quizzes and videos. The last of these are increasingly popular, but it is important that they are seen to be relevant to the workplace where they are shown. Some organizations make their own, and may run management competitions for the best one made.

The last British medical inspector of factories, Sir Thomas Morison Legge, propounded a number of aphorisms which are much quoted by occupational physicians. Among these are the following, all of which apply to this day (but to working women as well as men):

- Unless and until the employer has done everything, and everything means a good deal, the workman can do next to nothing to protect himself, although he is naturally willing enough to do his share.
- If you can bring an influence to bear, external to the workmen (that is, one over which he can exercise no control), you will be successful; and if you cannot, or do not, you will never be wholly successful;
- All workmen should be told something of the danger of the material with which they come into contact and not be left to find out for themselves– sometimes at the cost of their lives.

Education and training should not of course be confined to the shop floor, but should be provided at all levels in the organization. Uninformed managers and company directors are a far greater hazard than are uninformed workers, since their decisions may result in the loss or saving of many lives. In Britain in recent years, management ignorance of workplace hazards has become a serious problem.

6

Work-related accidents

Summary

Accidents at work are a commonplace problem, and their decline in frequency in Britain reflects more a change in the emphasis of work from manufacture to service and from male to female than a substantial increase in safety consciousness of the workforce. Accident rates in heavy industry remain unacceptably high, the worst offenders being mining, coke production, metal manufacture, railways and construction. This chapter summarises the relevant statistics in the United Kingdom.

Accidents generally arise from a conjunction of a hazard and an unsuspecting person. Machines, like people, have an inherent tendency to go wrong, while people may misunderstand or misuse them, or may be distracted. Accident prevention depends on attacking both causative factors, designing safer workplaces and machines, educating managers and workers in safe practices, and reinforcing those messages by safety audits. While the responsibility is primarily managerial, doctors and nurses in industry may play an important role.

Doctors and nurses also have responsibilities in training and ensuring the standards of first aiders and in planning for the immediate management and transfer of casualties. In hazardous industries, doctors in industry should liaise with local hospitals in planning for the management of major disasters. Doctors should also be aware of regulations with respect to reporting accidents and of the value of accident statistics, and should be able to advise their patients on appropriate methods of seeking compensation for accidental injury. These practical issues are discussed in this chapter.

Introduction

Accidents, which may be defined as unexpected occurrences usually involving injury or damage, are an experience common to us all. The attention of the media is attracted by serious, particularly fatal, accidents especially if they are of a sensational nature. Such episodes, involving loss of life or major damage to property, are of course the tip of a very large iceberg. Fatal accidents attract publicity related more to their unacceptability to society then to their frequency – for example, death from a railway or aeroplane accident (all rare events) are consistently reported in all national papers and on television; deaths from murder (around 600 per annum in Britain) are equally widely reported yet deaths in industrial accidents (400 per annum), deaths in traffic accidents (approximately 5,500 per annum) and deaths in domestic accidents (approximately 5000 per annum) are usually only reported in local newspapers, unless, as in the case of an oil rig explosion, they are part of a particularly major episode.

From the above figures it can be seen that death from a workplace accident in Britain is relatively uncommon. Such deaths have declined from about 1500 in 1961, to just under 1000 in 1970 to around 500 in the 1980s but rose to 730 in 1988/9 when 167 deaths occurred in the explosion of the Piper Alpha oil platform. This decline has occurred in spite of a rise in the size of the British labour force, (mainly attributable to a substantial rise in the numbers of self-employed) from about 25 million in 1971 to 28 million in 1990. Over that same period, there has been a relative shift in employment from industrial to service sectors (Table 6.1) and towards increased employment of women, and these factors have undoubtedly contributed to this favourable trend in that fewer people are engaged in the traditionally dangerous jobs.

Table 6.1 Employees in different industrial sectors (thousands)

	1971		1981		1990	
	Employed	Self employed	Employed	Self employed	Employed	Self employed
Males	13726	1556	12562	1641	12050	2449
Females	8413	397	9331	417	10806	773
Manufacturing	8065	129	6222	146	5151	272
Service	11627	1199	13468	1274	15868	1981
Other*	2447	625	2203	638	1836	969

Note * Agriculture, energy and construction

For purposes of data collection, it is necessary to define certain types of occupational accident that require to be reported. Every country has its own system, the only consistency being in the reporting of fatal accidents. In Britain, the following accidents are reportable under the Reporting of Injuries, Diseases and Dangerous Occurrences Regulations 1985 (RIDDOR, see Chapter 4):

- a death arising out of a workplace accident
- a major accident, defined as a fracture of skull, spine, pelvis or a long bone, amputation of a hand or foot, loss of sight in an eye, or any accident requiring overnight admission to hospital

- injuries resulting in absence from work for over 3 days
- episodes, such as leakage of explosive gas, explosions and collapse of stuctures, that had the potential to cause major injury but did not.

These Regulations probably ensure consistent reporting only of the most serious accidents, those requiring a night in hospital or several days off work often going unreported. Bearing this in mind, some figures are given in Table 6.2.

Table 6.2 Accidents of different severity 1986-91

	1986/7	1987/8	1988/9	1989/90	1990/1
Fatal	499	558	730*	475	410
Nonfatal major	22351	33804	33710	21706	20958
Over 3 days	160040	161011	164622	167109	158660
Fatal and major (per 100,000 employed)	100.8	95.7	93.8	93.4	90.1

Note: * Including 167 deaths in Piper Alpha explosion

These figures illustrate the considerable toll taken by workplace accidents, even though there appears to have been a slow decline in the rate of major ones in relation to the numbers employed. This decline may again simply reflect changes in the pattern of work rather than more effective preventive measures.

It is well known that some industries are more hazardous than others. These differences are clearly reflected in accident statistics, and figures for selected major industrial sectors are given in Table 6.3.

Table 6.3 Reported accidents in different industrial sectors 1990/1

	Fatal	Non-fatal major	Total	Rate/100,000
Coal extraction	12	541	4777	5478
Food, drink and tobacco manufacture	12	1177	14663	2805
Metal manufacture	5	351	3284	2132
Construction	93	2894	19377	1877
Chemical industry	5	494	3858	1212
Mineral manufacture	10	402	3646	1853
Transport	43	1440	16206	1207
Mechanical engineering	13	752	5830	791
Health services	–	689	9574	674
Agriculture	19	406	1542	636
Banking and finance	6	288	1746	66

The industries with the highest overall rates of reported accidents, all with a risk of over 2 per hundred people employed per annum in Britain (1990/91), are coalmining (5.8 per cent), coke ovens (2.9 per cent), other mining (2.3%), metal manufacture (2.1 per cent), railways (2.2 per cent) and food, drink and tobacco manufacture (2.8 per cent). Water supply, opencast coalmining and energy supply all have rates of 1.8–1.9 per cent per annum. The safest, unsurprisingly, are insurance and business services (approximately 40 per 100,000); it is interesting to note that agriculture, which has relatively large numbers of fatal accidents, seems to have a lower overall rate than work in health services; this almost certainly reflects under-reporting of less severe accidents in an industry where almost half the workers are self-employed. Similarly, the disproportion between fatal/major and total accidents in the construction industry is likely to result from under-reporting of the less severe.

Behind these figures lies an unquantified number of unreported and minor accidents. In a survey carried out by one of the authors, it was estimated that almost one in every 10 workers employed in the manufacturing industry and the agriculture/forestry/fishing sectors attends a hospital accident department each year for a work-related injury. Among these, some industries have very high rates of specific injuries – for example, in mechanical engineering, as many as 6 per cent of those employed suffer an eye injury requiring hospital attention each year. In the survey it was found that over 16 per cent of new attenders at the major regional accident department and almost 22 per cent of attenders at the corresponding eye casualty department had work-related injuries. However, because of its overall size, the service sector provided the largest total numbers of casualties of the major industrial sectors.

These figures give some idea of the importance of occupational accidents, both to the economy of industry and nations and also to the health of the population. This chapter considers the role of doctors in the workplace in prevention and management of the problem.

The causes of accidents

While dictionaries define accidents as 'unforseen' or 'unexpected' events, this should not be taken to mean that they are unforseeable. Their immediate causes are as varied as are accidents themselves, but ultimately, almost all can be traced back, with the advantage of hindsight, to the coincidence of two factors: an unexpected hazard and an unsuspecting human being. Appropriate action can reduce the risks from both factors. Although the science of risk assessment can produce estimates of the likelihood of events ranging from a worker tripping up and breaking a wrist to that of a jumbo jet crashing onto a nuclear power station, there nevertheless seems no limit to the ingenuity used by man to outwit such predictors.

Case history 6.1

The exploitation of nuclear fission for peaceful means has long been controversial, and designers of nuclear power stations have gone to great lengths to forsee possible system failures leading to major incidents. As far as possible, fail-safe systems have been built in to prevent the frightening consequences of an uncontrolled reactor melt-down. The first accident in the United States, which fortunately did not lead to loss of life, occurred when a worker was checking some wiring. Because the light was poor, he used a candle, ignited the inflammable coating of several wires, and put out of commission a major series of control and safety systems. The risk estimates had understandably not forseen the use of a candle, but might have been expected to have predicted the risk of fire when electric cables were coated with inflammable material.

Unsuspected hazards

The greatest opportunities for accident prevention arise from the recognition of hazards. Some physical hazards are extremely obvious – scaffolding, holes in the ground, cables strewn across floors, moving machinery and poorly stacked materials, for example. Many become more hazardous as a consequence of a second factor – ice on steps, water on floors, strong winds when working at heights. Poor lighting and noise can mask danger signs and increase risk. All these are relatively easily predictable, and sensible precautions to reduce risk can be taken.

Rather less obvious is the hazard entailed by breakdown of systems. All complex systems, including human beings, have within them a force tending towards disorder, known as entropy. This is demonstrable in people and animals by increased mortality and morbidity in the early stages and towards the end of life. In machines, for example cars and aeroplanes, the same phenomenon is observable with the highest risks of accidental breakdown being early and after several years of use. It may be kept at bay in machines by regular servicing, a benefit not available to animals (save possibly the humans who receive replacement joints or organ transplants). The natural lives of machines are as predictable in general as those of human beings, as are the likelihoods of breakdown of their various components. Thus it is possible to predict risks of accident due to such breakdown, although this process becomes extremely complex when systems comprising multiple inter-reacting structures and machines, such as an oil platform or a nuclear power station, are to be considered.

The keys to avoidance of a hazard are to appreciate its presence and to take appropriate avoiding action. Again this has two components – action by the person responsible for the presence of the hazard, such as the factory manager or the owner of the building, and action to avoid risk by those subjected to the hazard. Thus the risk imposed on individuals by a hazard is critically dependent upon individuals' perception of that risk and action taken to avoid it. Ultimately, when the engineer has completed the processes of designing and building the workplace, the machine or the system, risk depends on factors associated with fallible, often careless, human beings.

Case history 6.2

On the day he retired, the consultant cardiothoracic surgeon left his office to find that a hole had been dug outside his door to explore a defective drain. No warning notice had been posted and the hole was unprotected by a guard rail. Fortunately he saw the hazard and avoided falling into it.

What would you have done had it been you?

Understandably, he was annoyed by what he had found. He returned to his office and, being unable to contact the hospital manager by telephone, dictated a sharp letter to him, pointing out the possible consequences of such careless workmanship.

This anecdote will be continued in the next section, where we consider human factors in accident causation.

The unsuspecting human being

Accidents to people occur, by definiton, when the person does not appreciate the risk. Many factors may contribute to this lack of awareness. Among the more important are the following.

Gender

In general females are less liable to accidental injury than males. Almost 90 per cent of fatal and 78 per cent of other reportable industrial injuries occur in males, even though the numbers employed are roughly equal. Of course, men tend to select themselves into more hazardous jobs, but even in the same industrial sectors, the gender difference persists (Table 6.4). While some of this difference may be related to the fact that, even here, women have the less physical jobs, it seems likely that women take fewer risks than men and generally behave more sensibly.

Age

It might be thought that the young are at greater risk of industrial accident than the older worker, as is clearly the case with respect to traffic accidents. Younger people tend to be less experienced, somewhat more impetuous and perhaps to have a greater fear of appearing cowardly and a greater tendency to show off. However, although the numbers of reported accidents are greatest in younger employees, when these are corrected for numbers employed in the respective age groups there appears to be little difference (Table 6.5).

When age and gender are considered together, there is a tendency for male accidents to peak in the 25-34 year age group and female in the 45-55 year group.

Table 6.4 Accident rates per 100,000 in different industrial sectors, 1988/9

	Agriculture	Energy	Manufacturing	Construction	Services
Fatal					
Males	8.7	51.3*	2.6	11.3	1.4
Females	2.5	–	0.1	–	<0.05
Major					
Males	176.7	310.8	177.6	321.7	68.7
Females	81.6	40.4	64.6	23.0	35.6
Over 3 days					
Males	582.4	3400	1317	1842	723
Females	252.2	338	568	88.7	242

Note: * including Piper Alpha

Table 6.5 Industrial injury rates per 100,000 employed, by age and severity, 1988/9

Age	16–24	25–54	55+
Approximate numbers employed	6.2 m	17.3 m	3.4 m
Fatal	1	1	2
Major	53	60	48
Over 3 days	357	443	370

Industrial sector

Certain industries, as shown before, have high accident rates. While part of this is due to the intrinsic dangers of the work, there is little doubt that careless behaviour is characteristic of some sectors. This is particularly marked in the construction industry, where neglect of safety precautions such as wearing hard hats or safety harnesses, and failure to shore up the sides of trenches are responsible for many serious injuries each year. Such behaviour speaks of poor training and supervision of a workforce that is often transient and particularly insecure in its prospects of continuing employment.

Psychological problems

Concentration on the job in hand is clearly important at work, and any factors reducing such concentration may contribute to accidents.

Case history 6.2 (continued)

> The surgeon was enraged by the carelessness of managers in allowing the hole to be dug outside his office without warning or barriers. The episode caused him to think back over the many other battles he had fought with the hospital authorities over his career. Distracted by such thoughts and the emotions generated by his retiral, he hurried out of his office, fell into the hole and broke his ankle.

Episodes like this are probably more common than is realized. Family disputes, financial worries, depression and anxiety can all distract the minds of people at work and contribute to increase in risk from a hazard. Alcohol and drug abuse will have similar effects, and in the workplace the effects of hangover are well recognized as influencing accident liability. Lunchtime drinking will impair the efficiency of a manager; it may prove fatal to a worker exposed to moving machinery. Fatigue is particularly important, and this is reflected in regulations to limit the hours worked by lorry drivers and aeroplane crews. Somewhat belatedly, the importance of this is now being recognized with respect to hours worked by junior hospital doctors. Shift work has attracted a lot of research with respect to fatigue and causation of accidents, with rather inconclusive results. It should be remembered by senior managers that rotating workers between day and night shifts is analogous to regular aeroplane flights to the Far East and back. If the manager has been heard to complain of jet-lag, then the situation of the workers may be appreciated. It would be expected that effects of shift work on accident rates would be related to fatigue resulting from loss of sleep and disturbed circadian rhythms.

The concept of accident proneness has also attracted research, but it is difficult to see a useful, practical outcome from this. In the unlikely event of such individuals being detectable at pre-employment examination, their exclusion from the workforce at risk would be likely to make no appreciable impact on accident statistics, while excluding many who would never have had an accident (see Chapter 5, page 133, for analogy with exclusion of atopics).

Management factors

Managers make the biggest contribution to accident causation. All accidents are in theory preventable, by appropriate design of the workplace and the tasks within it, and by education and training of the workforce. Even when these steps are taken accidents occur when corners are cut to speed up a job or to facilitate it. When a company is under financial pressure it is likely that this pressure will be transferred down the line, mistakes will be made and accidents will increase.

Case history 6.3

A young man was working at a machine which compressed a mixture of two powdered metallic substances placed in a crucible. All such machines have a guard, which prevents access of hands into the press when it is being operated, and an interlock switch which prevents the machine being operated when the guard is open.

During the summer holiday period the factory was short-staffed and this coincided with the need to fulfil an order to a tight timetable. The operator found he could keep to his schedule more easily if he over-rode the interlock switch, allowing the guard to remain open during the compression. In putting the crucible into the press, he caught his fingers and required amputation of a terminal phalanx.

It may be seen from a case like this what opportunities are presented to lawyers, where a worker may blame a manager and a manager the worker. Both clearly contributed, the most important consequence being the lessons learned with respect to future prevention.

Communication failures

Failure of communication between people themselves, or between them and the machines or control rooms that they operate, is at the heart of many accidents. Avoidance of such failures lies in the realm of ergonomics (Chapter 5). Failure may, for example, be a consquence of noise obliterating a warning signal, of incorrect or no messages passed from a manager or colleague to a worker, of a worker failing to understand a badly designed dial, or of a broken or defective signal. Well-known examples include railway train crashes and the *Herald of Free Enterpriser* capsize; minor such episodes occur in workplaces daily.

The role of the doctor in prevention and management of work-related accidents

The prevention of accidents, or indeed the prevention of disease, is not primarily a medical matter. Doctors, by virtue of special training in the cauation of *diseases* are able to play a leading role in advising government, the general public and individual people on their prevention. In contrast, most doctors do not have a special understanding of *accident* causation (and hence prevention); rather we have confined our attention to the management of accidents once they have occurred, both by emergency treatment of individuals and by coordinated medical management of major disasters. Thus, other specialists have developed interests in accident prevention, the study of which has become of academic and practical interest to, *inter alia*, psychologists, engineers and ergonomists. In particular, responsible industries usually employ specifically trained safety managers, and national organizations exist in many countries for training and certification of those concerned with safety in the workplace.

In accident prevention, therefore, the doctor usually has only the role of other educated and sensible laymen. However, the doctor working in industry will often assume a more active role, related to knowledge of particular hazards of the specific industry, study of accident statistics and some expertise in the human factors related to accident causation. This may include, for example, examination and exclusion from hazardous work of people with conditions such as epilepsy, diabetes or alcoholism that may put them or others at increased risk. In most industries, accident prevention should be regarded as a team effort, with managers, trade unionists, safety officials and health professionals of various sorts contributing. In general, the leader of the team would be expected to be a manager with special knowledge of the hazards of the workplace. The doctor's advisory role would depend on what particular expertise he or she possessed. The doctor working in industry does, however, have a more significant role in the management of accidents. This includes training and maintaining the standards of first aiders (although this may be the responsibility of nurses or other appropriately trained people), the planning and implementation of methods for the immediate management of injuries, and ensuring that legal requirements for accident reporting are observed. Some large or particularly dangerous workplaces may have their own medical centre with a fully equipped accident department. Most have a first aid room. The doctor (or nurse) working in industry would normally be responsible for supervision of any treatment centre other than the most basic first aid facility.

Management of accidents

The doctor working in industry has a number of responsibilities with respect to accident management. These may include first aid provision and training, immediate medical care, documentation, reporting and, of course, planning for prevention. The doctor should also be involved in planning a strategy for dealing with major incidents in those workplaces, such as chemical factories or nuclear reactors, where such episodes are possibilities.

Dealing with the major incident

This is clearly the responsibility of senior management, but the doctor will usually have an advisory role in planning and a facilitatory role in the event of the accident. Plans will be specific to the particular worksite, and must forsee the possibility of explosion, fire, release of clouds of toxic gas or radioactivity, and multiple casualties. Detailed analysis of possible worst-case scenarios will be necessary, and appropriate action planned in conjunction with the local fire and police services, local hospitals and the ambulance service. Hospitals in the vicinity of hazardous industrial sites should be aware of possible injuries or gassings that might occur and should incorporate these possibilities into their major accident plans. The doctor in industry would be wise to assist local hospitals in running simulations of such accidents in cooperation with local authority services.

First aid provisions

In Britain, regulations govern the provision of first aid in the workplace, and the Health and Safety Executive regulates the training of first aiders; these are discussed in Chapter 4, page 82.

Over and above these provisions, the doctor working in an industry where there is a risk of particular accidents, such as poisonings or gassings, should make arrangements for immediate treatment on site, including administration of oxygen and antidotes if appropriate. Contact should be made with the local accident departments to inform them of possible emergencies and, in the case of risk of chemical poisonings, there should be ready access to the manufacturers' data sheets, which give the chemical constituents, medical hazards and first aid measures that may be necessary in the case of poisoning.

Case history 6.4

A chargehand in a petrochemical plant was responsible for injecting dimethyl disulphide from a container into an oil pipeline. This was done simply by turning on a tap which released the liquid chemical under pressure into a hose connected to the pipeline. On one occasion, as he did this the hose ruptured and he was sprayed all over with the chemical. The chemical has a distinctive, extremely unpleasant smell. He managed to turn the tap off, but had to walk 200 metres to the first aid post where he was stripped and showered. By this time he had become short of breath, and oxygen was administered, while the data sheet was being found. This said that dimethyl disulphide was a respiratory irritant and it was therefore concluded that respiratory support for possible pulmonary oedema might be needed. He was transferred, breathing oxygen, with the data sheet to the local hospital, where he was detained overnight and appeared to make a recovery. Subsequently, however, he developed persistent shortness of breath due to steroid-resistant airflow obstruction, and was thought to have suffered an obliterative bronchiolitis.

In general, the first aid management of industrial accidents is straightforward, involving support of vital organs and transfer to hospital, taking care to avoid making matters worse by inappropriate treatment. The management problems in hospitals come not from trauma but from poisonings, and the availability of a data sheet giving the name of the chemical and its adverse effects is a great help. In such cases, one of the national poisons centres may be contacted for advice. Even so, in many cases the best management of such rare episodes (as in the example quoted) is not known. In the case of acute respiratory irritants, there is anecdotal evidence that early administration of corticosteroids may reduce the risk of later obliterative bronchiolitis.

Reporting and investigation of accidents

In Britain employees have a duty, under the Health and Safety at Work, etc. Act, to report to their employer accidents resulting in any injury; the employer in return is obliged to keep an accident book in a prescribed format. Details of the individual, the events surrounding the accident and action taken are recorded. If the employee claims industrial injuries benefit, the employer has to make a return to the Department of Social Security.

As stated at the beginning of this chapter, accidents requiring a stay in hospital or more than three days off work, or involving major injury, are reportable by the employer under the Reporting of Injuries, Diseases and Dangerous Occurrences Regulations (RIDDOR), to the Health and Safety Executive. Deaths, major injuries and specified dangerous occurrences must be notified immediately by telephone and this must be followed up by written notification on a prescribed form. Other accidents requiring hospitalization or more than three days off work should be reported in writing as soon as practicable.

The reporting of an accident should not be the end of the process. All reports should result in investigation and preventive action. Both should be based on the matters discussed previously under accident causation. The investigation should take place as soon as possible after the event and should involve interviewing the victim (if possible), witnesses and supervisors or managers, and visiting the site of the accident. While it is a management responsibility, it should be made clear that its primary objective is not to apportion blame but to obtain information necessary to prevent recurrence. In the case of serious reported accidents, the Health and Safety Executive may well also investigate the circumstances and, if the employer is thought to have been in breach of the provisions of the law, a prosecution may result. In general, however, the objective of all such investigations is prevention of future episodes. Serious accidents should always result in the production of a report detailing the steps to be taken in this direction.

Keeping statistics

At factory, industry and national levels, statistics on frequency and severity of accidents are valuable indicators of the effectiveness (or lack of it) of preventive measures. The two components of interest, numbers of accidents and their severity, need to be related to the numbers at risk and the length of time over which people are at risk in order to give sensible information to managers when, as is usually the case, the size of the workforce fluctuates over time. The severity of accidents may be recorded by categorizing different types of injury or by recording indices such as hours or days lost from work.

Prevention of accidents

It should be clear from the foregoing that prevention of industrial accidents depends on an awareness of the fallibility of people, the dangers of machinery and workplaces and the risks inherent when the two interact. Prevention thus depends on ensuring as far as possible that the workplace is safe, that people in it are constantly aware of hazards and take active steps to reduce risk, and that systems are set up for regular safety checks or audit.

The greatest responsibility lies with management, who should normally include in their number someone with special responsibility for safety. But individual workers must also be made aware of their duties for the safety both of themselves and of their colleagues. Under the terms of the Health and Safety at Work, etc. Act, workers may nominate their own safety representatives, who should carry out regular safety inspections and report problems in writing to management, usually via the safety committee. Managers also should be responsible for regular audits of safety.

Setting up safety committees and appointing safety representatives is not in itself sufficient. The representatives should receive formal training, as should any managers with safety responsibilities, and all workers should be made aware of the importance of safe working practices and of action necessary to reduce risk. Dangerous areas should be clearly labelled and access restricted as far as possible, and machinery should be equipped with guards and other appropriate safety devices. Ultimately, it is the awareness by individuals of risk and their willingness to avoid actions that might have dangerous consequences that is the area where the greatest impact can be made in preventing accidents. Individual, often apparently quite trivial, acts of carelessness may have disastrous consequences.

Case history 6.5

Paper manufacture involves passing the fibrous pulp between pairs of very large rollers arranged in series. Access to the rollers is necessary in order to service them and to deal with tears or folds in the paper, but such access occurs only when the rollers are stationary. The platform allowing access is guarded by a rail and clearly labelled 'no access when machinery is running'. Nevertheless, on one occasion an experienced operator climbed over the rail to help feed the paper between the rollers while they were working, by kicking at it. He slipped on the wet floor, his foot was caught in the machine and his body was delivered in fragments moments later.

This horrifying story is repeated, with minor differences, every month in workplaces throughout Britain. It emphasises the need for safety training to be taken seriously by everyone. Management should have a written safety policy and should set an example themselves by always wearing appropriate safety equipment, such as boots and eye protectors, in designated places.

There is much scope for originality and initiative in devizing safety training and promoting safety awareness in an organization. Safety fairs, videos and quizzes with prizes all have more impact than lectures or written information. Incentives, such as safety bonuses for parts of the organization with least accidents, need to be used with care, however, as they may result in a failure to report injuries. In all these activities, the occupational physician or nurse, with their knowledge of the consequences of accidents in terms of human suffering, can play an important role.

Compensation for workplace injury

In Britain, two different systems are available for an injured worker to seek financial compensation. Both are discussed more fully in Chapter 4. Under Industrial Injuries legislation, people injured at work (except the self-employed) may claim disablement benefit if they are suffering loss of physical or mental faculty 15 weeks after the injury. Faculty means the ability to perform at the expected level of someone of the same age and sex. For payments to be made, and these are additional to normal invalidity benefits (see Chapter 7), the loss of faculty must be assessed by an independent panel of doctors as at least 15 per cent.

In addition to industrial injuries benefit, an injured worker may sue the employer in the civil courts for negligently causing injury. The verdict is usually made by a judge sitting without a jury, after hearing the arguments by counsel for both parties and cross-examination of expert witnesses. As may be imagined, the process is often prolonged and costly, and many cases are settled on a 'no liability' basis out of court. Workers are generally supported by their trade union or out of public funds. If the action is successful, the State in Britain is able to obtain refund of injury and other Social Security benefits paid, out of the court settlement.

In the United States, the preferred option is usually to seek retribution in the civil courts, where plaintifs' lawyers can, and frequently do, take cases on a speculative basis, taking no fee if unsuccessful but sharing in the settlement if the case is won. These cases are heard before a jury, who not only decide the verdict but also determine the size of the award. While in Britain this is generally determined on the basis of compensation for pain, suffering and loss of earnings, in the United States the option open to the jury of adding a large sum for punitive damages has made many lawyers rich!

7

Sickness absence

Summary

Control of sickness absence is the responsibility of management. However, the presence of a mild or moderate degree of ill health alone does not necessarily mean that the affected person will take time off work. Other factors of which managers should be aware may make a significant contribution to absence levels.

A distinction must be drawn between persistent, intermittent short-term absences which are not linked with a consistent medical condition and where an employer may argue 'substantial reasons for dismissal' and genuine long-term acute or chronic sickness absence. In the latter case there is a duty on management to seek alternative employment where a return to the original job is impossible (see Chapter 8). Where there is a residual disability the employer will be required to consider making minor modifications to the original job to aid the employee's return to work particularly where there has been a contributory industrial injury or occupational disease.

For managers to make fair decisions they must demonstrate that they have acted 'reasonably' and have sought the appropriate medical advice. However employers are not expected to create a vacancy nor can it be assumed that the employee would be prepared to take any particular job. The employer may eventually have to terminate employment under the heading of 'Capacity', i.e. ill health.

Persons who are unable to work because of ill health may be entitled to a range of social security benefits. The payment of statutory sick pay is a contractural obligation of the employer who determines, for his organization, for how long payment will be made. Many employers will pay more than the national rate of sickness benefit through contractural arrangements with the employee. If employment is terminated because of continuing ill health, the patient will then receive sickness benefit from the Department of Social Security if the requisite number of National Insurance contributions have been made. Sickness benefit is, therefore, a contributory benefit available for the first 28 weeks of certified sickness absence. Invalidity benefit is a contributory benefit which is payable for periods of incapacity lasting over 28 weeks.

Doctors have a duty to be aware of the benefits available, where information can be obtained, and how their patients gain access to the system. They also have a duty to provide supporting medical evidence where required. This is particularly pertinent to benefits related to disablement which are discussed in detail in Chapter 8.

Introduction

The health assessment of workers in relation to sickness absence forms a substantial part of the work of most occupational physicians. It also presents a dilemma to general practitioners who may have to balance the actual health status of their patient and fitness to work against the patient's self-perception of readiness to return to work and associated financial and social considerations.

Case history 7.1

A 55 year-old female domestic assistant was referred to the occupational physician by her manager. She had returned to work 2 months after surgical repair of a femoral hernia. Her manager was concerned that she was not able to carry out her full range of duties. Discussion with the patient revealed that she had pain and intermittent discomfort in the appropriate iliac fossa which was exacerbated by lifting and stretching. She had not been able to undertake her normal household duties including vacuum cleaning but in spite of that, and against the advice of her general practitioner and physiotherapist, she had insisted on returning to work. She felt guilty at being away for so long when she knew that the hospital were unable to employ any temporary help to cover her absence owing to financial constraints. Physical examination revealed a well-healed scar but surrounding tenderness and discomfort when raising her head and shoulders off the couch and 'stressing' the muscles of the anterior abdominal wall. Enquiries into her range of duties showed that she was required to do high level and low level dusting, mopping and buffing of floors, emptying rubbish pails and nappy pails and clearing away and washing up cooking utensils.

During the consultation she burst into tears admitting that she was not ready to come back to work. The occupational physician wrote both to her manager and general practitioner stating that she would not be fit to return to work for at least a further month.

The principal outcomes of sickness absence are shown in Fig. 7.1.

This chapter discusses the contributory factors associated with sickness absence, which are complex and multifactorial, the management of the immediate problem and benefit entitlements. Rehabilitation, retirement on medical grounds, disability and the employment of the disabled are discussed in Chapter 8.

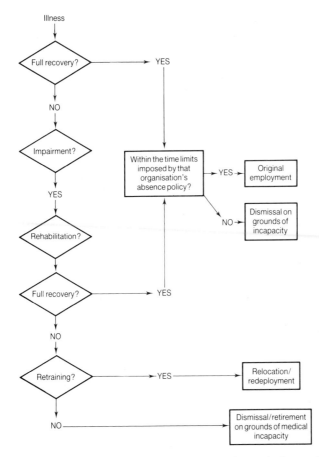

Fig. 7.1   Outcomes of ill health in relation to prospects for continuing employment

What is the size of the problem?

The cost of sickness absence to the British economy was estimated at £5.5 billion in 1987. This does not take into account the hidden costs which may be summarised as:

- overtime to cover for absentee
- temporary help to replace absentee
- supervisory time spent to find a person to cover absence
- lowered morale and decreased productivity of those remaining at work, particularly if part of a small interdependent workforce
- 'catch-up time' required by returning absentees.

Every year in Britain, on average, 3 weeks per employee (8% of available work time) are lost due to ill health. This includes all types of sickness absence ranging from self-certification to long-term absence. There has been a gradual rise over the years from 300 million days lost in 1964, to 361 million days in 1982/3, to 472 million days in 1989/90. It should be noted that these figures do not take into account changes in the total size of the workforce in employment which had changed over this period and therefore a more accurate comparison can be made if the figures are expressed as days lost per 1000 employees, Table 7.1.

Table 7.1   Days lost due to ill health

Year	Days lost (millions)	Size of workforce (thousands)	Days lost/ 1000 Employees
1964	300	24882	12057
1982/3	361	23348	15462
1988/9	433	26173	16543
1989/90	472	22864	20644

The most recent figures are based on claims for sickness and invalidity benefit with men contributing 338.5 million and women contributing 133.2 million days. These figures ignore absences of less than 3 days which do not require self-certification and absences of less than 8 days which are self-certified. It has been calculated that 1–3 day absences account for approximately 15% of sickness absenteeism.

Ill health resulting in sickness absence may be as a result of work related illness, for example, occupational asthma, many forms of dermatitis and upper limb strain disorders; personal ill health, for example, cardio-vascular disease, diabetes; or an interaction between the two, for example many cases of low back pain and psychological breakdown. It encompasses both physical and mental illness. As we shall see later there are other relevant contributory factors.

Diseases and injuries caused by work are all theoretically preventable by identifying and assessing the risks and following the hierarchical sequence of appropriate preventative measures as required by the COSHH Regulations (see Chapter 5). To put these measures into practice requires communication with managers, unions, employees and, at the individual's level, with the general practitioner. As we shall see, communication is equally important when evaluating the effect of personal ill health on the ability to work. Moreover, the workplace offers the opportunity for prevention and education not only regarding work related ill health but also morbidity resulting from lifestyle factors such as smoking and alcohol consumption (see Chapter 9).

The common causes of ill health absenteeism

Work Related Ill Health

Musculo-skeletal Conditions

While these conditions affect a large number of people it is often very difficult to assess the occupational contribution both individually and overall. It has been said that the affected individual is in many ways the best placed to make this judgement! Nine to 10 million people are employed in occupations likely to involve a significant amount of manual handling. Nearly half of all adults of working age will experience some low back pain in any 6-week period. In Britain in 1982/3 33.3 million working days were lost due to back pain which contributed 9.2% of the annual certified sickness absence at an estimated cost to the NHS of £168 million and lost production in excess of £1000 million. In 1991, the number of working days lost was 46 million and the cost in medical treatment, sickness benefits and lost production was of the order of £1.75 billion. Currently back injuries result in 52 million lost working days annually, 12% of the total. In the United Kingdom back pain and other musculo-skeletal problems are the most common causes for referral to an occupational physician.

Under the RIDDOR Regulations (see Chapters 5 and 6) there were 150,000 reportable injuries in the United Kingdom in 1988/9. Musculo-skeletal injuries contributed 41.6% overall, see Table 7.2, and 27.5% of reported accidents involved manual handling.

Table 7.2 Musculo-skeletal injuries reported under RIDDOR 1988/9

Type of Injury	Nature of Work	Number
Sprain/strain	Handling, Lifting, Carrying	35000
Sprain/strain	Other causes	24000
Upper limb strain disorder	Repetitive Work	3500
Total		62500

It is known that only a percentage of reportable accidents are reported. The 1990 Labour Force Survey, conducted by the Office of Population, Census and Surveys estimates the level of musculo-skeletal injuries for that year, including upper limb disorders, at over 650,000. Musculo-skeletal disorders in general are the most common cause of absenteeism due to work related ill health not only in the United Kingdom but throughout the Western hemisphere.

Respiratory Disease

Past exposure to high levels of dusts in the workplace is still contributing to work related ill health. In the United Kingdom over 1,000 new cases of disease due to past exposure to silica, coal dust and asbestos are awarded disablement benefit each year. In 1988 there were 1324 deaths attributable to occupational lung disease. The contribution of occupationally related asthma to sickness absence is increasing. Some 500 cases of occupational asthma are being reported annually in Britain and this probably represents a three-fold underestimate.

Occupational Dermatitis

In 1980/81 there were estimated to be nearly 100,000 cases annually of occupational dermatitis in Britain. In 1989 the figure was about 60,000. Many of these patients are unable to work at the job that provoked the disease and thus skin disease is a significant and largely preventable cause of sickness absence.

Occupationally Related Cancer

In a review of the number of 'avoidable' cancers, that is, cases where removal of the workplace exposure would have led to avoidance of the cancer, it has been estimated that 4% of cancers (range 2–8%) could be avoided by the elimination of all workplace carcinogenic risks. Of these, asbestos has been the major factor and thus this proportion may fall appreciably as a result of control measures now in place in the developed world.

Personal Ill Health

It is difficult to draw a clear line between the various factors contributing to a particular category of disease. Over the years there has been a decline in deaths due to infections and respiratory disease while deaths due to cardiovascular disease and cancer have risen. The principal causes of work time lost in 1989 in relation to diseases of non-occupational origin are heart disease, respiratory disease, cardiovascular disease and breast cancer with heart disease, for example, accounting for 62 million work days lost per annum in the United Kingdom in 1988/89. Some of these conditions may also have work related factors ranging from exposure to chemicals and fumes, to stress. It has been suggested that 16% of premature deaths from cardiovascular disease in Denmark could be prevented by workplace intervention.

Many employers intuitively feel that people with chronic illnesses such as diabetes or epilepsy will have substantial sickness absence. This preconception is discussed further in Chapter 8. However, such conditions are not the bar to employment that many recruitment managers suppose. It is a pre-requisite that the condition should be well controlled on appropriate medication, that there are no work-related factors, such as working at heights which would automatically bar an epileptic, and that the patient is under regular medical supervision. Each applicant should be assessed as an individual. Thereafter it has been shown that employees with a chronic disability do not have excessive absence rates and frequently have a lower than average sickness level. As we shall see in Chapter 8 many people with severe disability can continue to work effectively with the full use of resources for the disabled.

Mental illness contributes significantly to the role of personal ill health in absenteeism and is frequently the result of a combination of work related and domestic factors. Psychiatric, psychological and other mental health problems, including stress, rank second following musculo-skeletal disorders with regard to the number of referrals to occupational physicians in the United Kingdom. Approximately 40% of all sick leave is believed to be due to minor psychological ill health, and job dissatisfaction may play a major part. Treatment may be lengthy and there is frequently a need for rehabilitation and integration back into the workplace to restore confidence and thereafter effective performance. Inevitably, in some cases the outcome is less than satisfactory.

Case history 7.2

A 25 year-old man, married with two young children, developed panic attacks following the sudden death of his mother. Although he was given treatment by his general practitioner the frequency of the attacks increased and inevitably he experienced an attack at work although there was no specific work-related trigger factor. He was sent home and became severely agoraphobic, afraid to leave the house or to travel on public transport in case he had a panic attack. Treatment was continued with a combination of medication, psychotherapy and physiotherapy to teach breathing techniques. He gradually improved over a 4-month period, became able to leave the house, but not able to travel on public transport. He felt he could cope with his job as a warehouse supervisor but could not travel unless he had a car ride with his father; unfortunately that did not coincide with his shifts. Management agreed that initially his working hours could be rearranged to allow him to have a lift with his father and, as he continued to improve, he was eventually able to use public transport and resume shift working. However his total absence from his contractual employment was 8 months.

His return to work was short lived and, after 6 months, he again had a recurrence of severe anxiety and a panic attack at work. He felt that on this occasion it was triggered by pressure of work which was contributed to by staff shortages and increased demand prior to Christmas. Discussions with the manager showed that there was no possibility of alleviating either of these trigger factors. The general practitioner referred him for further relaxation therapy and exercises to prevent him hyperventilating. The psychiatrist changed his medication but the tablets had significant side-effects which he was unable to tolerate. The occupational physician undertook a domiciliary visit and discussed the possible outcomes of this lengthy period of sickness absence. The patient agreed that the occupational physician could write to his psychiatrist for a report and also draw his attention to the fact that the entitlement to paid sick leave would be expiring within 6 weeks and the most likely outcome would be termination of his contract on health grounds. The psychiatrist was asked to consider whether there was any further line of treatment which he felt would be helpful.

The occupational physician and the patient were pessimistic about the final outcome; the patient because he felt that all avenues of treatment had been explored and he had been unable to make a sustained return to work previously despite attempts to facilitate this by changing his working hours and restructuring his duties. The occupational physician was aware that there were no further treatment options and that management were not convinced that the patient would ever be able to contribute effectively in the workplace. The patient was retired on health grounds. However, he and his family were optimistic that he could make a 'new start' elsewhere.

Contributory Factors

Reasons for sick leave are often complex and influenced by non-medical factors. The levels of absenteeism may be associated with factors such as age, gender, personality, domicile, working conditions and sickness benefits.

Age   Sickness absence increases with age, see Fig. 7.2, but patterns differ. The below 20s have a higher frequency of short duration absence particularly

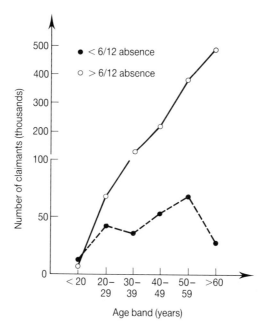

Fig. 7.2   Number of claimants (thousands) of sickness and invalidity benefit in relation to age and duration of absence

in the first 5 years of employment. This relates to a new environment, totally different from the familiar ones of home and school; the need to learn new processes and techniques; integration into a team and acceptance by colleagues who may no longer be a homogenous peer group. Absence is used as a coping mechanism for stress. Longer term absences increase markedly with age, reflecting the onset of more serious ill-health.

Gender   A survey of 10 different occupations found that absence rates were consistently greater in females than males. This may relate more to domestic and social responsibilities than illness. The statistics on invalidity benefit, published by the Department of Social Security, show a higher number of claimants for sickness/invalidity benefit in women under 30 years compared with men, which correlates with the ages of maximum reproductive capacity and young families. Overall, as shown in Fig. 7.3, there are fewer women claimants than men when the figures are standardised for the numbers in employment.

Personality   Much attention has been paid by recruitment officers to matching personality to job demands. Psychological assessment, aptitude tests and even more speculative techniques such as handwriting analysis and astrological forecasts have been employed to fit 'round pegs into round holes'. There is no

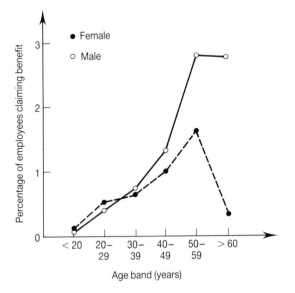

Fig. 7.3   Percentage of employees in employment claiming sickness and invalidity benefit in relation to age and gender

doubt that mismatch between job requirements, particularly where team work is involved, can lead to dissatisfaction which may be manifested as sickness absence.

Geographical   There are significant differences in absence rates between regions of the United Kingdom. For example, Wales has a rate 50% higher than the average while the absence rate in South East England is lower than average. This may in part reflect regional differences in types of industry, for example, the more manual the nature of work the higher the level of absence.

Work Organization   It has been said that working conditions may be more important that social and demographic factors in influencing absenteeism. Relevant factors are dull, unrewarding employment with low status which may be hazardous, stressful and physically demanding. Unskilled workers have three times the sickness rates of managerial grades. The size of the work group has been shown to be important. The larger the group, the more anonymous each individual becomes. Re-organization into small groups where each worker has responsiblity for a particular component of the end product has been shown to raise morale and self-awareness and reduce absenteeism. The feeling of being welcome and needed is important and the attitude of the departmental manager may be influential in determining whether a sick employee makes the effort to go to work.

Case history 7.3

A 28 year-old single man had worked as an operating theatre porter for 8 years. He developed back pain following a lifting injury and was referred to the occupational physician who referred him for physiotherapy. He was absent from work for 4 weeks. He returned to work for 2 weeks only to have a recurrence of his symptoms which necessitated a further 5 days absence. Ten days later he developed an upper respiratory tract infection and although unwell came into work after visiting his general practitioner only to be told by his manager, 'I don't know why you bothered to come in, you're no use when you are here anyway.' His sickness absence level increased significantly. He was referred to the occupational physician.

During the consultation it was established that he had intermittent pain and discomfort following his previous episode of back pain. Whereas previously he had gone to work he now took 1–2 days absence. Assessment of his back showed no significant impairment of function and the cause of his absence was clearly related to managerial attitudes. The occupational physician in discussion with senior management was able to arrange for his relocation. Thereafter his sickness absence record improved substantially.

Economic   The company's sick pay scheme, the length of employment and the number of hours worked per week may all inter-relate in determining the length of sickness absence. Organizations which provide fully paid sick leave for 6 months followed by half paid leave for 6 months may know from experience that some employees will return when their fully paid sick leave entitlement expires independent of their health status. Part-time low paid workers, for example domestic and catering staff in the NHS, may even be financially better off on sick leave as their statutory sick pay may open the door to additional benefits (see later) increasing their income to greater than that when at work.

Indices of sickness absence

How do we define absence levels? Before being able to participate in the 'management' of sickness absence, the occupational physician must be aware of the parameters that prevail within the organization. There must be a clearly defined base line applicable to all departments at which intervention takes place so that there can be no accusations of favouritism. The following indices can be used to quantify absence:

Prevalence Rates

Point prevalence: $\dfrac{\text{no. of people absent on a day}}{\substack{\text{total population of workforce} \\ \text{who should be present that day}}} \times 100$

Period prevalence: $\dfrac{\text{no. of people absent over a given time}}{\substack{\text{total population of workforce who should} \\ \text{be present during the given time.}}} \times 100$

Severity

Lost time per cent: $\dfrac{\text{hours work time lost due to absence}}{\text{expected normal working hours}} \times 100$

Average annual duration per person:

$$\dfrac{\text{total days lost/person due to absence in year}}{\text{* expected normal working days}} \times 100$$

* The expected normal working days must be defined for any particular organization as they may vary from

- calendar days   – 365
- work days   – 312 (based on 6-day working week)
               – 250/235 (taking into account holiday entitlements)

National Insurance statistics are based on a work year of 312 days.

Frequency

Average length of absence spell: days absence

number of spells

Inception rate: total number of new spells per annum

population at risk

The distribution of absence periods in the workplace, as shown in Fig. 7.4, is frequently skewed. In general, half the total time lost is caused by 5–10% of the workforce. However, research has suggested that the frequency of spells of absence is increasing rather than duration. The prediction of frequency of absence levels among individuals relates most closely to their record in their first year of service.

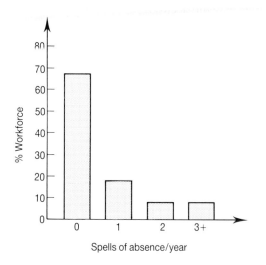

Fig. 7.4   Distribution of absence spells in workforce

Categories and management of sickness absence

Absence may fall into one of three categories:

- uncertified – absences less than 3 days.
- self-certified (Form SC1) – absences lasting more than 3 but less than 8 calendar days.

- medically certified (Form MED3) – absences 8 days or longer.

Sickness absence of interest to managers usually separates into recurrent short-term or long-term, either acute or chronic. In either category the people may not necessarily be sick, there may be non-medical reasons. It is therefore common for managers to receive either no certificate or self-certificates in recurrent short-term absence whilst long-term absence may commence with a self-certificate but will subsequently be medically certified. Managers must take the responsibility of monitoring absenteeism and guidelines (see list below) have been laid down by Employment Appeal Tribunals as to what steps employers must take to show that they are acting reasonably and have sought appropriate medical advice.

1. The employer must investigate the facts, review the attendance record and reasons for absence. Reports and/or recommendations from the occupational physician should also be reviewed to ensure that relevant advice has been implemented wherever is reasonably practical. Any underlying coherent pattern should be identified.

2. The employee's explanations must be considered.

3. The employee must be warned under the disciplinary procedure that the level of absenteeism is unacceptable, the attendance record must improve and within what time limit. Also the employee must be told what will happen if there is no progress.

4. The employer must consider an appropriate penalty, for example a written warning or dismissal, and treat each case on its merit. If all intervention fails, dismissal may be the final and inevitable outcome.

These steps will be influenced by the pattern of absence.

Recurrent Short-term Absence

Employees with bad records of recurrent absence should be formally interviewed by management. Many large organizations identify 'trigger' points for action when an individual record approaches either the national average or a pre-set accepted level for the individual organization. Using such a scheme managers may also be seen to be acting impartially and avoid charges of victimization. Examples of 'triggers' are:

- 4 separate spells of self-certified absence in a rolling 12 month period, or
- 14 days of self-certified absence in a rolling 12 month period (whichever happens first), or
- frequency factor
  $$- \text{number of days} \times (\text{number of spells})^2$$
  $$\text{e.g. } 9 \times (3)^2 = 81$$

with a pre-set action level of 20.

However, use of impersonal parameters can induce further problems.

Case history 7.4

One large organization arbitrarily introduced a sickness absence monitoring programme without informing the occupational physician or ensuring that the changes were communicated to the employees. All employees with more than 12 days absence in a 12-month period were interviewed by personnel managers regardless of the diagnosis or cause of the sickness absence. They were then referred to the occupational physician for 'confirmation' that the diagnoses were genuine and required the associated amount of sick leave despite appropriate certification from the general practitioner at the time of the absence. Needless to say this caused anger and resentment among staff who felt they were being accused of malingering. Morale and motivation dropped and some felt that their jobs were threatened.

The interview should identify for the individual employee whether recurrent short-term absences are due to a clearly identifiable underlying medical problem or, alternatively, whether the information on absence certificates poses, to the manager, a variety of seemingly unrelated diagnoses. It is not appropriate for the manager to pry into confidential medical matters and, at this stage, referral to the occupational physician may be appropriate. The basis of the referral and the role of the occupational physician must be clearly understood by all parties.

Referral may be formal or informal and formal referral will require a formal report. Employees must be reassured at the beginning of the consultation that it is confidential and the overriding aim is to provide help or support. Any report to management will not divulge medical information unless it is essential, in the interests of health and safety, and even then it will not be divulged without the informed written consent of the employee. However, the occupational physician has an important role to play in advising management about the prognosis, when the employee would be likely to return and whether redeployment should be considered. The report will, therefore, give an opinion on the patient's fitness to work. The processes involved in decision-making are listed in Table 7.3. The issue of confidentiality is discussed again later in this chapter

Table 7.3 Factors in decision making

Define problem	–	attendance		
	–	capability		
Gather valid information	–	job	–	description
			–	absence record
			–	accident reports
	–	clinical	–	history
			–	physical examination
			–	investigations
			–	review past records
			–	consult other involved professionals
Process information				
Formulate advice	–	further absence		
	–	rehabilitation		
	–	redeployment		
	–	retirement		
Communicate advice	–	personnel		
	–	line management		
	–	employee		
Evaluate outcome	–	improved attendance		

following case history 7.6. The outcome of any referral may be positive or negative.

Formal Referral

Consistent History

The following letter was received by the occupational physician.

Case history 7.5

Dear Doctor
re: Name   D.O.B.
       Address

Please will you arrange to interview and examine, if appropriate, the above second year student nurse whose sickness absence record is giving cause for concern.
The attendance record for the past year is:
- medically certified days absence   16
- self-certified days absence   21
- uncertified absence   5

                                                         Total   42

The diagnoses have been sinusitis/tonsillitis.
I would be grateful if you would ascertain

1. Whether there is any serious underlying medical condition to account for this absence record.

2. Whether the absence record is likely to improve in the future. The allowable sickness absence during the training period is 3 weeks.

She is agreeable to being referred to yourself.

Yours sincerely,
Tutor

This constitutes a formal referral and therefore a written report is expected. The referral letter might also have included more specific details regarding the job, for example, physically arduous, mentally stressful, involving shift work, even though the occupational physician would be expected to routinely enquire into these areas. The manager might also have noted whether there was any pattern to the absence, for example, related to days before and after leave entitlement, weekends, or start and termination of shifts. Reference must also be made to the Access to Medical Reports Act, 1988, and the employee consulted as to whether he/she wishes to see the report before it is sent to the manager. The application and ethical aspects of this Act, in relation to occupational medicine, are discussed in Chapter 10.

> The patient attended the Occupational Health Department, rather aggressively, saying that she had 'always had sore throats and sinusitis and had been told nothing could be done'. She managed her symptoms by having 'the odd day off' and only seeing her general practitioner if she felt she needed antibiotics. Her doctor therefore had no knowledge of the extent of the disruption to her training and she, until interviewed by her tutor, had not realised how much absence had accrued.

If you were the physician to whom this patient had been referred, what approach would you take? Clearly it is necessary to obtain a detailed account of the job, with factors such as shift patterns, difficulty with tutors and fellow students enquired into. Secondment to other hospitals, with temporary accommodation, ought to be taken into consideration. Information about social factors such as late nights, problems with parents or friends, alcohol consumption are also important. An appropriate medical history and examination are always essential.

> The medical history indicated that she had an uncomfortable and unpleasant recurrent infective problem. This was confirmed by the findings on examination of facial pain over the maxillary and frontal sinuses and large, fleshy tonsils. No investigations had ever been undertaken. Communication with the general practitioner suggested that sinus X-rays might be helpful and availability of the occupational health department, to monitor the frequency of symptoms and origin of infection from throat swabs was accepted.

The report to management confirmed that Jayne had a contributory underlying medical condition, stated that she had been referred to her general practitioner for investigations and that referral to a specialist would follow if the results of the investigations and monitoring of her symptoms by the occupational health staff warranted it.

Monitoring showed a consistent pattern of recurrent infection with haemolytic streptococci. She was referred for tonsillectomy. Subsequently her sickness absence was minimal.

This case had a successful outcome. However, almost identical referral letters with a similar clinical history, have resulted in negative findings on examination and from investigations. In such cases the offer of monitoring the symptoms may also lead to their rapid and virtually complete resolution together with attributable absences. Equally, in other cases, social or interpersonal difficulties may seem to be responsible for the repeated absences and the resolution of the problem may lie more in the hands of the manager.

Inconsistent History

Case history 7.6

A woman, aged 50 years, had worked for the Health Authority for 20 years as a clerk in the Supplies Department. Stores and supplies were re-organised on a regional basis 3 years prior to her referral. Contracts of employment, at the time of re-organization, had been changed from district to regional level. Computerization was introduced together with bulk buying. Staffing levels were rationalised. The patient began to take time off work with increasing frequency, a day or two here and there with 'indigestion', 'backache', 'gastro-enteritis', 'migraine'. In other words a pattern of recurrent short-term absence with no coherent underlying cause. She was referred to the occupational physician.

She recounted the changes in organization which had occurred and which she felt had resulted in loss of identity for members of the department. They had previously been part of the hospital 'team' with direct contact with ward sisters and department managers who knew they could rely, in times of crisis when running short of essential supplies, on a personal response. There were increased complaints from 'users' at the rigidity of the new system. As well as this depersonalization there was unfamiliarity with new technology systems which had been introduced. Rationalization of staff levels led to an increased workload with responsibility for both processing orders and dealing with complaints. Having been previously recognised and respected as competent and helpful she now felt 'useless' with loss of self-esteem and the development of stress-related symptoms.

What would you do? Two complementary approaches were indicated, first to help the patient and second to ameliorate the working conditions.

Coping strategies were discussed. These included a discussion of relaxation techniques to practice both in the workplace and at home, the importance of discussing her feelings and frustrations with both her general practitioner and her husband and involvement in leisure activities such as walking. In respect of work she was advised that she must always take her lunch, coffee and tea breaks away from the office so that she would not be distracted by the telephone ringing and feel that it ought to be answered. She agreed to see her general practitioner taking with her a letter from the occupational physician outlining the work-related symptoms. On the other hand, management were alerted to the contribution of the work environment to the problem but, as often happens, were unable to implement any tangible changes.

The situation temporarily improved but she later presented as a long-term sickness absence referral having had a recurrence of stress-related symptoms which she described as difficulty in getting to sleep at night because of worry as to whether she had correctly entered the orders, early morning wakening and worrying about the day ahead with particular fears as to whether she would have to deal with any abusive telephone calls. She lost her appetite and consequently lost weight. She lost interest in her hobbies and found it difficult to cope with visits from her daughter and grandchildren. Despite further treatment from her general practitioner and formal referral for stress management, relaxation and coping techniques it became clear that she was not going to make a permanent recovery within that working environment. There were no opportunities for redeployment and she was eventually retired on grounds of a chronic anxiety state which rendered her unable to carry out her duties.

The role of the occupational physician in rehabilitation and redeployment is discussed in Chapter 8.

Inconsistent diagnoses contributing to a pattern of short-term recurrent absences may also reveal an underlying problem with substance abuse, particularly alcohol, or social problems. Information from the manager regarding the pattern of absence and associated factors such as lateness, accident levels or changes in work performance may provide clues as to useful lines of enquiry.

Informal Referral

A manager may suspect there is an underlying problem affecting work performance and attendance before the 'trigger' for formal interview has been reached but wishes to intervene at an early stage. Referral very often takes the form of a telephone call from the concerned manager who, having interviewed the employee, realises there is some sort of health related problem but the employee is unwilling to be formally referred.

The stigma which still surrounds any diagnosis of mental ill health such as anxiety/depression is a common reason for employees declining formal referral and for general practitioners putting ambiguous diagnoses on medical certificates. Employees are anxious that there should not be reference on their personnel record to any factor which might affect prospects for promotion or references for future jobs.

Case history 7.7

A 50 year-old man, divorced and living alone, was a senior manager with day-to-day responsibility for the efficient running of an organization employing 2,000 people. He was noted to be having increasingly frequent short-term absences and a pattern emerged that these were on days when he should be attending meetings or submitting reports and also after return from annual leave. There had also been reports of inappropriate behaviour in meetings with tremor and slurred speech and an occasional smell of alcohol. After a great deal of persuasion he agreed to talk informally to the occupational physician where, it transpired, he was on medication for hypertension and insomnia. He admitted to anxiety prior to giving presentations which manifested itself as tremor, and quickening and slurring of his speech. He vehemently denied alcohol abuse.

Should the occupational physician have persisted in trying to confirm the implied abuse? Should consent for liver function tests have been sought? What if consent was refused?

The patient agreed to consult his general practitioner for stress counselling and coping strategies. He also agreed to allow the occupational physician to talk to his senior manager and confirm that there was 'an underlying health problem' for which he was receiving appropriate medical treament. The attendance and behavioural problems improved in the short term but then recurred and it became clear that this was the start of a long term problem.

Nine months following the first referral, the occupational physician received a telephone call from the senior manager. The previous pattern of frequent short-term absences, inappropriate behaviour in meetings both 'in house' and in public had recurred and again there were hints of alcohol misuse. He was interviewed by his managers and the occupational physician was asked to see him but he immediately commenced certified sickness absence before an appointment could be arranged. The diagnosis was stress and anxiety. Shortly after the commencement of his absence numerous empty bottles of spirits were found by chance in his office.

How should the occupational physician proceed? To wait until he returned to work would provide no opportunity for discussing rehabilitation schemes both in terms of his own personal health and in relation to the work environment. In addition, the confidence of the senior manager, in the patient's ability to be able to return to a job that would continue to be stressful, was lacking.

After the first month's absence, the occupational physician approached the general practitioner to ascertain whether the patient was responding to treatment and when the general practitioner felt it would be appropriate for the occupational physician to contact him to make a preliminary assessment as to when he might be able to discuss the work situation. The general practitioner consulted with his patient and it was agreed that he was well enough for a domiciliary visit to be undertaken. During the visit the patient admitted that he had a longstanding alcohol problem for which he was now attending group therapy. It became clear that although he was making progress he was certainly in no fit state of mind to make any rational decision as to what his future employment options might be. However, the range of possible options, which included 1) return to his original job, 2) relocation within the organisation, 3) retirement on health grounds were broached, and it was agreed that the occupational physician would review the situation with the patient in a further month. The patient was reassured that whatever the outcome no final decisions would be made until he was mentally well enough to make a rational decision.

Absence due to underlying psychiatric problems and/or substance abuse is difficult to evaluate both for the occupational physician and the manager. Until the employee has the confidence to admit the true underlying cause treatment may be inappropriate and therefore ineffective. Obviously, once the true diagnosis is admitted, the employee must be:

- re-assured that his illness and resulting absence will be treated as any other and in accordance with the workplace policy (ideally the workplace will have a specific Alcohol at Work Policy with emphasis on treatment and rehabilitation – see chapter 9, p 219).
- encouraged to give consent for his/her manager to be informed and, providing the above reassurances have been given, this is usually forthcoming.

It must not be forgotten however that where consent to divulge such information is refused and there is a conflict, in terms of health and safety, between the cause of the ill health, e.g. alcohol misuse and the occupation e.g. driving, the occupational physician has an over-riding duty under the Health and Safety at Work etc Act to inform management of the situation.

Role of Management

Occupational health staff can, therefore, help to evaluate the reasons for short-term repetitive absences purportedly due to illness. The history is important, physical examination may be unproductive, evaluation of social, domestic and emotional factors is mandatory. Job-related factors such as poor interpersonal relationships and supervisory attitudes should be conveyed to the appropriate managers with the consent of the employee. If all intervention measures and implemented recommendations fail to improve the absence record the employer can fairly dismiss having followed the guidelines laid down by the employment appeals tribunal which were described earlier in this Chapter.

Non-medical reasons for absenteeism

It can be difficult to distinguish these from 'genuine' sickness absence. Two employees with the same medical diagnosis and objective physical and/or functional impairment may have vastly different sickness absence rates. In this situation discussion between the occupational physician and the employee may reveal either work related factors, for example, the employee does not like the job or there are interpersonal conflicts with colleagues or supervisors or there may be relevant social or domestic factors.

Case history 7.8

A 24 year-old shift porter, had frequent uncertified absences and persistent lateness on the morning shift. When he was at work it was agreed that he performed at an above-average level. Informal referral to the occupational physician, to which he agreed, elicited the facts that he was the oldest of 5 children all living at home and that his mother suffered from chronic ill health. One of his younger sisters was abused by an older member of the family and although her bedroom door was locked at night his sleep was disturbed by the slightest noise. He felt that he needed to be at home if she was alone in the house, for example, at weekends. When his mother was unwell he was responsible for getting the youngest children to school.

Further enquiries into what avenues of help or advice had been sought, such as the general practitioner and social worker, were unproductive as he insisted that he would not discuss the family situation in any greater detail.

Although it was suggested that recommendations could be made that he left shift work, he insisted that no report should be sent to his manager other than agreeing that 'there was no underlying health problem contributing to his absence'.

Although in absenteeism, no formal medical investigation is necessary, there must be a fair review of the attendance record and the reasons for it.

In this case, warnings of the likely consequences if there was no improvement enabled the employee the opportunity to give an explanation. However, he did not volunteer any further information and, as might be expected, was finally dismissed.

Long-term absence

When dealing with long-term ill health absenteeism the employer must take the following vital steps:

- Try to discover the true medical position with respect to severity of the illness, likely time off work and likelihood of return to work. The manager is not entitled to ask for confidential medical details.
- *Consult* with the employee regularly.

- Allow the employee a reasonable length of time in which to recover.
- Consider alternative employment within the organisation.

The situation must be weighed up bearing in mind the employer's need for work to be done and the employee's need to recover his/her health.

If the employee refuses to attend the occupational health department and it is not a condition of employment, initial informal counselling by the occupational health staff with regard to reassurance of both clinical confidentiality and the employee's access to medical reports may be effective in bringing about a change of mind. It is not uncommon for the employee to see referral to the occupational physician as a threat to employment rather than the first step in, whenever possible, achieving either a satisfactory return to work or redeployment. Referral to the occupational physician will also take into account the company's arrangements for paid sick leave and ill-health pensions. Those organisations which provide paid sick leave for 6 or 12 months may not require a formal referral to the occupational physician until 3 or 6 month's absence has elapsed, particularly if there is a well-defined underlying cause such as a major surgical procedure. However, communication between managers, general practitioners, consultants and the occupational physician is essential to achieving the optimum outcome for the employee.

The referral letter to the occupational physician from management must set out very clearly the duties of the employee. The occupational physician should have good knowledge of the workplace and already know what those duties are but, if further information is required from the general practitioner or consultant, identification of the duties forms an essential component of the request. The letter must also state what information the employer requires.

Example

Dear Doctor,
re: Name   D.O.B.
    Address

Mrs X has been employed as a full-time/part-time (number of hours) domestic assistant at the Royal Infirmary for 4 years. Her duties involve high and low level dusting, sweeping, mopping and floor buffing, washing up, cleaning sanitary ware, making and serving patients' tea.

She has now been absent for 2 months with a diagnosis of (for example) arthritis. I have interviewed Mrs X and she is agreeable to being referred to you.

I would be grateful if you would let me know
  1.   The likely date for a return to work.
  2.   Will there be any residual disability.
  3.   If so will it be temporary or permanent.
  4.   Is he/she likely to be able to render regular and efficient service in the future.

5. Is there any requirement to consider
   (a) a period of rehabilitation
   (b) redeployment either temporary or permanent.
If so please include any restrictions or limitations that are appropriate.

Yours etc.
Manager

Difficulties may arise when the general practitioner/hospital consultant considers that the patient is fit to return to work but the manager/occupational physician disagrees or vice versa. Where the general practitioner and occupational physician disagree managers will generally prefer the opinion of the occupational physician who should be more knowledgable of the workplace environment and its effects on health. The occupational physician will be able to balance the fitness or well-being of the patient with the demands of the job, as illustrated in case history 7.1, and will also take into account the method of travel to and from work and the design of the workplace. All these factors are relevant and are discussed further in Chapter 8.

Benefits

Doctors, whether in primary care, or occupational health practice, should be able to provide patients with information as to what benefits are available and how to claim them. They should know that leaflets are available in the local Department of Social Security Office now called the Benefits Agency, at Citizens Advice Bureaux and local authority information centres. Local authorities employ welfare rights officers who are usually located at the Town Hall but, in some areas, may be seconded to work within the district hospitals. Many aspects of Social Security benefits are linked to ill health and disability and their availability to patients is dependent on the statutory role of the doctor in providing supporting medical evidence.

Benefits may be divided into contributory, non-contributory and means tested as shown in Table 7.4. Sickness and invalidity benefits are discussed in this Chapter whereas in Chapter 8 disability living allowance, disability working allowance and severe disablement allowance are discussed in relation to rehabilitation. Industrial injury benefits are described in Chapter 4.

To qualify for benefit in relation to ill health a patient has to show that he/she is 'incapable of work by reason of some specific disease or bodily or mental disablement'. The cause of the condition does not have to be definitely identified and, whereas normal pregnancy does not count, conditions arising from it such as nausea, vomiting or hypertension are relevant.

Table 7.4   Benefits relevant to ill health

Contributory	Sickness Benefit
	Invalidity Benefit
Non-contributory	Industrial Injury Benefit
	Statutory Sick Pay
	Disability Living Allowance
	Severe Disablement Allowance
Means tested	Disability Working Allowance
	Income Support
	Housing Benefit
	Community Charge Benefit

Sickness Benefit

Sickness Benefit is paid for up to 28 weeks to anyone unable to work on account of sickness if that person has made the requisite number of National Insurance contributions. It is thus available to the contractually employed, the self-employed and some currently unemployed people. The responsibility of paying sickness benefit to those people contractually employed was devolved to the employer in 1983 with the introduction of Statutory Sick Pay (SSP). Under this scheme, although the employer may not pay less than the national rate of sickness benefit, many employers pay more through contractual sick pay arrangements. The occupational physician should be aware of employees' entitlements when considering the period of certification and the urgency of referral for specialist opinions or treatment such as physiotherapy. Initially a patient's incapacity is looked at in relation to the normal job. After 4–6 months the Department of Social Security (DSS) will begin to consider whether the patient is able to do alternative work. This will also depend on factors such as whether the patient's original job is being held open, the likelihood of recovery in the near future and the proximity of normal retirement age.

Invalidity Benefit

Invalidity benefit is paid for periods of incapacity lasting over 28 weeks when patients have already received sickness benefit or statutory sick pay for 28 weeks. There is an age related addition termed invalidity allowance.

After benefit has been paid for several months the recipient may be referred by the DSS to a doctor from the Regional Medical Service. This is particularly common in respect of absence due to chronic back symptoms but other conditions also 'trigger' the process.

Case history 7.9

A 55 year-old senior administrative assistant developed chest pain and fatigue in 1984. Her symptoms began 12 months after her husband underwent coronary artery by-pass surgery and subsequently required a considerable amount of care at home. They also coincided with increased responsibilities at work coincident with lack of secretarial support. Her symptoms escalated and she was eventually admitted as an emergency to the coronary care unit where she underwent coronary angiography. Although this was normal her electrocardiograph (ECG) had abnormalities consistent with intermittent cardiac vessel spasm which was felt to be aggravated by stress. She was treated with sublingual glyceryl trinitrate.

Other than tiredness she remained relatively well for the next 12 months when she developed a sudden onset of extreme tiredness, nausea and vertigo coincident with exacerbation of her angina. During the 12-month period there had also been an increase in her workload due to reorganisation.

Discussions with her cardiologist led to him giving an opinion that no further medical treatment was indicated and it was decided that she would apply for early retirement on the grounds of ill health. This proceeded uneventfully. Six months later, while still on paid sick leave and awaiting finalisation of her pension she was referred by the DSS to the Regional Medical Service in respect of her invalidity benefit. She subsequently contacted the occupational physician at her place of work, in great distress, to say that her invalidity benefit had been refused on the grounds that she was capable of working.

What happens now?

It is important to realise that the Regional Medical Officer's opinion is not binding on the general practitioner who should continue to issue sickness certificates as considered appropriate. The general practitioner may well discuss the situation with the occupational physician at this juncture or the patient may request to see the occupational physician bemused by events – one doctor says she cannot work, another says she can! The DSS may then refer the patient to a second Regional Medical Officer; if this doctor concurs with the first, benefit will cease. If the general practitioner, knowing the patient, and the occupational physician, still consider the patient to be incapable of work they can help to convince the adjudication officer or Social Security Appeal Tribunal by writing a fuller statement as well as continuing to issue sickness certificates.

In the case of the senior administrative assistant an appeal was lodged with supporting evidence in the form of a report from the occupational physician which detailed her physical condition and medication with a description of the effect that that had on her ability to work. It highlighted symptoms such as lack of concentration, impairment of short-term memory and the onset of fatigue earlier than might be expected in a healthy woman of the same age. It was also pointed out that no interventional treatment was indicated and that her condition would not be improved by any change in her medical treatment. The appeal was successful and the patient continued to receive her invalidity benefit.

8

Rehabilitation and the employment of the disabled

Summary

Rehabilitation encompasses those medical and occupational activities which enable an ill or injured person to live independently and gain or regain the necessary skills for employment. Occupational rehabilitation must, wherever possible, proceed together with medical rehabilitation as part of a structured approach to a return to work.

The occupational physician has to assess the physical and mental state of the patient with regard to the functions which contribute to disability and balance that assessment against the requirements of the workplace. When a balance cannot be achieved the options of redeployment, retirement on the grounds of ill health or referral to specialist rehabilitation centres must be investigated.

A proportion of men and women of working age have a disability which handicaps them in terms of employment. However, disability does not equate with ill health. When their medical fitness for work is assessed, the task of the occupational physician is to relate the patient's condition, interpreted in functional terms, to the demands of the job.

Occupational physicians have unrivalled opportunities to provide the co-ordination between medical, social and vocational rehabilitation schemes and to facilitate the entry or return of those disabled or handicapped by disease, injury or accident into the work environment. Doctors in the workplace must be aware of the specialist services provided by Placing, Assessment and Counselling Teams and their Disability Employment Advisers; the range of financial and advisory services; and the provision of specialist equipment which is available to facilitate the employment of those with disabilities. Occupational physicians should also be aware of the Social Security benefits which are available for the disabled and be able to advise their patients as to how to obtain pertinent information.

Introduction

The preceding chapter discussed the role of the occupational physician in the management of sickness absence. One of the most important aspects in determining whether a worker will return to employment after injury or significant illness is assessment of the functional recovery. This chapter discusses the scope of such an assessment in relation to the potential for returning to work, the value of rehabilitation programmes and their availability and the range of possible outcomes. Disabled persons, whatever the source of the disability, are frequently disadvantaged both in obtaining and remaining in employment. The range of services available and financial benefits are discussed in the second half of this chapter.

Concepts and definitions

It is important that there is a clear understanding of what is meant by the different terms used in describing the sequelae of injury or illness. In 1980 the World Health Organisation proposed the following international classification of impairment, disabilities and handicaps (ICIDH).

Impairment is a change in normal structure or function resulting from a disease, disorder or injury. It encompasses any loss or abnormality of a psychological, physiological or anatomical structure or function. The disturbance is at the level of the 'organ', e.g. loss of a limb, hearing or sight. The result is a structural disablement.

Disability is any restriction or lack (resulting from an impairment) of the ability to perform an activity, e.g. climbing stairs, operating machinery, in the manner or within the range considered normal for a human being. It reflects disturbance at 'person' level, e.g. behaviour, performance, mobility, communication, memory. As a functional disablement it should be seen as a continuum in terms of severity, ranging from very slight to severe. This has importance in relationship to employment as progression of the disability may require further modifications and adaptation of the workplace to allow continuing employment, as will be discussed in case history 8.16.

Handicap is a disadvantage for a given individual resulting from an impairment or disability that limits or prevents the fulfilment of a normal role for that individual. That role may be in relation to a particular environment, e.g. work, and the consequences may be cultural, social, economic and environmental. They may be manifested as physical, in relation to independence; social, in respect of integration; and economic in relation to self sufficiency. Handicap is a restrictive disablement.

The above definitions can be illustrated by the following examples:

Case history 8.1

A 55 year old woman developed severe osteo-arthritis of the hip, the objective changes of loss of joint movement being an impairment causing lack of mobility. The resulting disability was the lack of ability to stand for any length of time, to walk any significant distance, climb stairs or drive. She was handicapped by being unable to continue working as a community nurse.

Case history 8.2

A 23 year-old kitchen porter had had chronic osteomyelitis of his foot for 8 years resulting in bone erosion and a limp, i.e. impairment. Due to the continued activity of the infection he had an elective below-knee amputation resulting in a disability in walking and climbing stairs and a major social and occupational handicap.

It must be noted that the definitions apply to both physiological and psychological illness and are not restricted to locomotor disorders.

Case history 8.3

A 55 year-old woman employed as a senior manager and researching into the development of paper record systems developed impairment of mental function by nominal dysphasia and physical function by right sided hemiparesis following repeated transient ischaemic cerebral attacks. In terms of disability she had a reduction in manual dexterity with reduced ability to write quickly or legibly and operate a keyboard. She was handicapped socially and occupationally by decreased concentration, poor short-term memory and nominal dysphasia.

The outcome in this case and in case history 8.2 will be discussed at various stages throughout this chapter in relation to assessment and rehabilitation.

Rehabilitation is the process of helping individuals to maximise their physical, psychological and social capabilities to cope with life, after they have, in some way, been deprived of their former capabilities.

Medical rehabilitation encompasses all activities which will enable a person to live independently. It will incorporate the skills of various health care workers, for example, doctors, nurses, physiotherapists, occupational/speech therapists and psychotherapists, and techniques such as reconstructive surgery and the use of technical aids. Both physical and mental activities must be encouraged at an early stage and be appropriate to the physical and mental capacity of the patient.

Occupational rehabilitation describes the activities to enable a person to gain or regain skills for employment. These activities may be workplace orientated and/or provided by government agencies such as Employment Rehabilitation Centres (ERC) or skill centres.

Resettlement defines those activities which enable a return to the previous employment or redeployment following the acquisition of any relevant new skills.

Occupational rehabilitation should commence as early as possible during recovery. It should not be seen as a sequel to medical rehabilitation but, wherever appropriate, as proceeding in tandem. The advantages are an increase in the morale and confidence of the patient and a decrease in apathy and boredom. Where there is an occupational health service, liaison should commence at an early stage between the occupational physician or nurse, the personnel and line managers, the employee and the involved doctors, be they the general practitioner or hospital consultant. Discussions can take place regarding the possibility of rehabilitation, the agreement to develop and participate in a programme, the appropriate time for its introduction and the means of evaluation. The agreement of the employee to participate may be influenced by outstanding litigation and compensation claims. In organisations or small industries where there is no occupational health service, the general practitioner may find it helpful, with his patient's consent, to directly approach the personnel or line manager and discuss the possibilities for an early, phased return to work. On the other hand, the patient who is a 'key' worker may be approached by his manager with proposals as to how an early return to work could be facilitated.

Assessment

The general practitioner or hospital consultant frequently has to answer the question from his patient, 'When can I go back to work?' Before making any decision, the physical and mental fitness of the patient must be balanced against the physical and mental demands of the job, adhering to the concepts that were discussed in Chapter 1. If the patient has had specialist treatment the general practitioner can liaise with the consultant during out-patient follow-up or may receive a discharge summary which clearly specifies how long it will be before the patient is fit to return to his normal duties. Obviously someone with a physically demanding job will require longer absence following a fractured femur, or herniorrhaphy, than a patient with sedentary employment. Conversely, a patient with a psychological illness such as anxiety or depression, who is in a mentally demanding job, will require a longer absence than one undertaking a routine physically orientated task. Any possible adverse effects of the job or work environment on the patient's health must also be considered.

Account must be taken of associated factors such as transport to and from work, the distance travelled, the physical environment of the work-place, for example, stairs, as well as the actual physical requirements of the job. A machine operator or assembly line worker may not be physically active in the wider sense but may have to walk a long distance or climb several flights of stairs to reach the actual point of work and then spend most of the working day standing. Shift work and the mental demands of interaction with colleagues and/or the public after a period of limited social contact must also be considered. It is in these areas that the occupational physician or nurse can provide relevant advice and collaborate with the doctors providing clinical care in facilitating a return to work. They must also be aware of the practical difficulties to be overcome in initiating a rehabilitation programme. These may relate to:

- personal problems confronting the employee, for example, the mental attitude to work following a life threatening event, lack of confidence in ability, fear of learning new skills.
- management attitudes, for example, inflexibility, ignorance of the potential abilities of an employee with disability or handicap, ignorance of the services available to facilitate rehabilitation (these are discussed later in this Chapter) and fears of a high level of sickness absence.
- financial restraints, for example, personal social benefits may outweigh the salary for part-time or low paid workers; there may be union-negotiated bonus schemes dependent on quotas being met or multidisciplinary working; or profits in small industries may be affected by a decrease in work rate or other similar contribution compared with colleagues.

Case history 8.4

A 40 year-old hospital domestic assistant had suffered from schizophrenia for many years. He coped well with his narrow, prescribed range of duties. Reorganisation led to amalgamation of domestic and portering services and the concomitant introduction of bonus schemes required job flexibility. The fear of having to work in different areas to cover sickness absence, the fear of dealing with patients as a porter and the overtly expressed views of his colleagues (who were normally very supportive) that he would reduce bonus payments led to increased morbidity and the request for early retirement on health grounds.

What approaches can you think of to tackling this problem? Is there any room for compromise?

With his permission, the occupational physician held discussions with the appropriate managers which resulted in an agreement that the patient would not be included in calculations for the bonus scheme and would continue to work as before but in a supernumerary capacity. He remained in employment and his sickness absence record and general well-being improved to its former level.

After a long absence the following questions should be posed:

- Has the employee's ability to carry out the job safely and effectively been affected with reference to self, other employees and, if appropriate, the public?
- Will the health of the employee be compromised by continuing in that work?
- Will the job, pattern of work or workplace have to be modified permanently or temporarily?

- If necessary are there facilities for continuing treatment (see case history 8.9)?

Assessment must therefore be in two parts, the person and the job.

Personal assessment

Table 8.1 lists 13 recognised functions which contribute to disability, that is, the restriction or lack of the ability to perform an activity in the manner or within the range considered normal for human beings, regardless of the pathological process.

In occupational rehabilitation attention must be directed to assessing those functions which will have a direct bearing on the ability to return to employment. The following case histories illustrate the relevance of the various functions in relation to work.

Table 8.1 Personal assessment of disability

Functions		Parameters
Locomotion	–	walking, climbing steps/stairs, bending and straightening, balance
Reaching and Stretching		
Dexterity	–	holding, gripping, turning
Seeing	–	distance/near
Hearing	–	tinnitus
Continence	–	bladder and bowel control
Communication	–	being understood, understanding others
Personal care		
Behaviour		
Intellectual functioning	–	memory, concentration
Consciousness	–	fits/convulsions
Nutrition and digestion		
Disfigurement	–	amputation, burns, cosmetic

Physical abilities

Case history 8.2 (continued)

Following his below-knee amputation, the 23 year-old kitchen porter was fitted with an artificial leg. Approximately one month later he was seen by the occupational physician who had already established with the personnel manager and the kitchen supervisor that every effort would be made to rehabilitate him back to work although both managers were highly sceptical of achieving a positive outcome.

In practical terms he was able to demonstrate that he could climb steps and stairs and had sufficient stability to achieve good balance which enabled him to twist and turn, reach and stretch. He did not yet have stamina to enable him to weight-bear or be physically active for any length of time. This was partly due to the continuing adaptation of the stump to the socket of his artificial limb. However, mentally he was very apprehensive about returning to work. He perceived himself as 'disfigured' and a freak and was unsure of the reaction of his colleagues. He was also worried about being pressurised into returning to work within a defined time limit.

The outcome of this initial assessment was the opinion that he would be able to return to work, with the minor reservation that he might experience irritation of the stump due to the heat and humidity in the kitchen, but that more time was required to allow his stump to adapt. He returned for a further assessment one month later. During the interval he had been visited at home by both the personnel manager and kitchen supervisor. This visit improved his self-esteem particularly when they stated that he was a valued member of the team and also removed any fears of being pressurised into undertaking any jobs before he felt confident to do so. He had also increased his own confidence in his abilities by decorating an elderly disabled neighbour's house.

At the second assessment he was full of confidence in his abilities and an individual rehabilitation scheme was implemented. This will be described later.

Dexterity

Case history 8.5

A 40 year-old firefighter lacerated his left forearm in a fall at home. This resulted in impairment through damage to his median and ulnar nerves with subsequently a complete degeneration lesion of his ulnar nerve at the site of the injury. This was confirmed by electromyographic studies. Clinically, there was wasting of his interossei and lumbrical muscles and loss of sensation along the medial border of the forearm and the fourth and fifth fingers. Nerve regeneration was detectable after four months.

He regained full movement of his left wrist and, in spite of loss of abduction and adduction in his fourth and fifth fingers, his disability improved in that he developed the functional ability to grip tools and manipulate equipment. The sensory loss in these fingers remained. A practical assessment of his functional capabilities on the fireground was undertaken satisfactorily and he returned to full duties.

Hearing

Case history 8.6

A 23 year-old firefighter sustained a severe head injury in an unprovoked assault. The outcome was total and permanent unilateral deafness and tinnitus. He was retired on health grounds.

Firefighters must have bilateral hearing to enable them to localise sounds, instructions and warnings.

Continence

Case history 8.7

A 40 year-old security guard had an ileostomy for ulcerative colitis. Assessment was required to ensure that he had physically recovered from surgery, his ileostomy was functioning predictably and he had the confidence and facilities to change ileostomy bags at work.

Communication/Disfigurement

Case history 8.8

A 55 year-old surgeon had a total laryngectomy and block dissection for carcinoma of the larynx resulting in considerable cosmetic disfigurement. He subsequently developed oesophageal speech.

At assessment, he related that he had already seen a small number of long-standing patients on an individual basis and now felt confident that his disfigurement was not a handicap and also that he could communicate adequately both face to face and over the telephone. This was confirmed by the occupational physician. As he still lacked physical stamina a rehabilitation programme in relation to a reduced work schedule was implemented but sadly he died suddenly 6 weeks after returning to work.

Personal Care

With developments in renal dialysis and the introduction of continuous ambulant peritoneal dialysis (CAPD), patients with renal failure whose renal function is maintained in this way may be able to return to work providing they are not significantly impaired by chronic anaemia. Treatment with erythropoietin may, in future, remove this obstacle as well in a proportion of cases.

Case history 8.9

A 30 year-old nurse on CAPD was assessed before returning to work in the endoscopy department. The facilities to change the equipment at work were provided together with the necessary time allowance. Although she had a significant anaemia she felt she could cope with the demands of the job and it was arranged that her ability to continue working would be monitored jointly by the renal and occupational physicians. She was able to remain in full-time work until a donor kidney became available when she underwent successful renal transplantation. At the time of writing she will be assessed three months post-transplantation with a view to resuming work following appropriate rehabilitation.

Behaviour and Intellectual Functioning

This is one of the most difficult areas to assess in relation to the ability to return to work and one where knowledge of the intellectual requirements of the job and the importance of interpersonal relationships is essential. Disability may be idiopathic, for example, Alzheimer's disease, may result from self inflicted damage such as abuse of alcohol or drugs, or may be the consequence of a head injury (which may or may not be work related) or of exposure to neurotoxins such as solvents.

Case history 8.10

A 40 year-old senior manager was unexpectedly exposed, over a period of three hours, to intermittent high levels of mixed solvents originating from paints and which could not be individually identified. The acute effects were severe headache, upper respiratory tract irritation and mild symptoms of narcosis. While the respiratory effects and narcosis resolved within 72 hours the headaches persisted. Over the next month, he underwent a significant personality change, becoming withdrawn and prone to violent rages. He was forgetful, unable to concentrate and unable to talk or write fluently with intermittent aphasia. Neuropsychological assessment at 6 months and 12 months post-exposure confirmed both personality and memory defects. Suggestions were made for rehabilitation programmes to modify behavioural responses and improve cognitive functioning. However, because of the requirements of his job in terms of both intellectual and personnel functions, he was retired on health grounds.

Consciousness

The assessment of someone who has had or has the potential to have fits or convulsions will depend on the existence of any primary cause, for example, tumour, and its treatment, the response to and compliance with anticonvulsant therapy and the requirements of the job.

Case history 8.11

A 40 year-old firefighter, whose individual role included driving fire appliances, had a brief episode of cerebral dysfunction including a transient hemiparesis and altered facial sensation. The putative diagnosis was an intracerebral bleed but cerebral angiography showed no obvious cause such as a berry aneurysm. The firefighter had no further clinical symptoms and his neurological abnormalities completely resolved within 2 weeks. Magnetic resonance imaging 6 weeks later showed a small area of scarring at the site of the bleed. He was referred to the occupational physician for assessment. His employers felt he was no longer fit for employment in the Fire Service. Physical examination was entirely normal and he was anxious to return to work.

The occupational physician had to balance, on the one hand, his excellent personal health and, on the other, a duty of care to the public in respect of the small possibility of the development of post-traumatic epilepsy which had been estimated by his consultant neurologist as less than 5 per cent. Expert independent neurological opinion was sought so that there was no bias related to personal care of the patient. The occupational physician was advised that freedom from fits for 12 months from the date of the original episode would place the risk of having a fit in the future at no greater than a fit occurring for the first time in a member of the general public.

The firefighter was very antagonistic to the occupational physician and provided letters from his specialist to support his immediate return to full duties. However, the occupational physician gave him the option of 12 months restricted duties, dating from the time of his intracerebral bleed and followed, if all remained well, by return to full duties, or retirement on health grounds. He chose the former option and having remained fit and well was fully resettled.

Attitude

Those who have had a life threatening illness or operation may feel that, having cheated death once, the most must be made of the rest of their life. Although thorough clinical assessment following rehabilitation may confirm physical fitness to return to employment, mentally the patient may not be prepared to accept any possible risk, particularly if it is felt that the original precipitating factor for the illness was work related. A common example is a high physical demand or 'stress' in relation to myocardial infarction. Although persuasion by the occupational physician may be initially productive in that the employee returns to work, this outcome might not be sustained.

Case history 8.12

A 62 year-old male domestic assistant sustained a myocardial infarction. He made an excellent recovery and, after assessment at 3 months post-infarction, he commenced a rehabilitation programme with restricted duties and shortened working hours. By 6 months post-infarction he had resumed normal, full-time duties. At 9 months post infarction he requested to see the occupational physician and asked to be considered for ill-health retirement. He gave a history of minor aches and pains but no significant disability and then said, 'I don't feel I should be working after a heart attack. I have had one chance and it is time to take life a bit easier'.

What would you do?

The occupational physician, after again reassuring him that his symptoms were not indicative of angina and offering him a further cardiological opinion, discussed with him, with the consent of his manager, the option of shorter hours and a lighter programme of work similar to that which he had undertaken during his rehabilitation programme. However none of these options were acceptable. He made it clear that he had already approached his general practitioner who was willing to furnish him with sickness absence certificates for the duration of his sick pay entitlement. At his age and with his past medical history he would be highly unlikely to obtain further employment and so he was retired, rightly or wrongly, on the grounds of anxiety secondary to his myocardial infarction.

Job assessment

The general characteristics of the individual's job should be confirmed to discover whether there has been any material change from those factors operating at pre-employment assessment. Such factors might be whether the job is skilled or unskilled, strenuous or light, paced or intermittent and whether there are any general or specific environmental hazards such as extremes of temperature or the potential for exposure to toxic substances. In particular, enquiries should be made about physical, sensory and intellectual requirements of the job, some of which are listed in Table 8.2.

The role of job assessment is illustrated by returning to the case of the senior records' manager with the transient ischaemic cerebral attacks.

Table 8.2 Assessment of job requirements

Physical	Sensory	Intellectual
Strength	Vision	Concentration
Endurance	Hearing	Memory
Mobility	Smell	Communication
Coordination	Touch	Comprehension
		Learning
		Decision-making
		Problem-solving

Case history 8.3 (continued)

At assessment to look at the opportunities to return to work or to make recommendations for redeployment, it became clear that this 55 year-old record systems manager had considerable intellectual impairment following her transient ischaemic cerebral attacks. Her concentration and short-term memory were impaired and she had intermittent nominal and receptive dysphasia which affected both communication and comprehension. Her ability to take quick decisions which might have far-reaching implications was impaired as was her ability to use computer systems safely. Because of her seniority it was felt that any available redeployment would not be appropriate and she was retired on health grounds, the intellectual requirements of her job being incompatible with her mental state.

Rehabilitation schemes

Following assessment, the range of options available for each individual is considerable as shown in Figure 8.1. They range from immediate return to normal duties at one end of the spectrum to ill health retirement at the other and include rehabilitation programmes in the workplace and referral to statutory agencies.

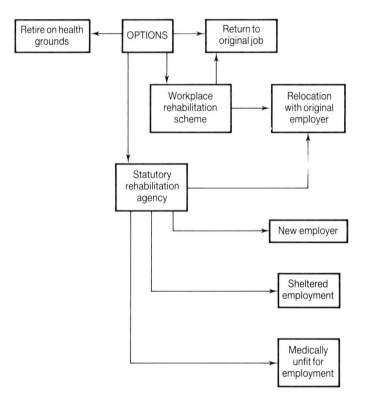

Fig. 8.1 Options following long term sickness absence

Workplace schemes

The aim of these schemes is either to return the employee to his original job or, if assessment during this period shows that this will not be achieved, explore, at an early stage, the opportunities available for relocation together with any necessary retraining. The options to consider are:

- immediate full time normal duties with assessment by the occupational physician or occupational health nurse after one month or sooner if necessary or

- full-time, 'light' duties for a specified time or
- part-time, 'normal' duties for a specified time or
- part-time, 'light' duties graduating to part time, normal duties and leading eventually to resumption of full time normal working.

'Light duties' implies avoidance of those activities which are likely to exacerbate or delay recovery from the presenting complaint. In terms of physical activities this requires, for example, avoidance of lifting, pulling, pushing heavy objects. With respect to mental function, the patient would be advised to avoid situations where instant decision-making was required or there was inevitable face to face confrontation with difficult clients. Each programme must be tailor-made for the individual and develop either the range of duties or the length of working hours in a gradual manner during the rehabilitation period. For example, recovery from back injury would require, principally, a reduction in the range of duties, while rehabilitation following an acute anxiety state is more likely to entail a reduction in working hours. A standard example is shown in Table 8.3.

Table 8.3   Scheme for part time working

Week	Monday	Tuesday	Wednesday	Thursday	Friday
1	–	half day	–	half day	–
2	half day	–	half day	–	half day
3	half day	full day	half day	full day	half day
4	full day	half day	full day	half day	full day
5–8	Normal day working				
9	Return to shift working if appropriate				

Any scheme, as discussed earlier in this chapter, must take into account personal factors, transport to and from work, avoidance of rush hour travel and both the organisation and scope of the work. This is exemplified by returning to the case of the amputee kitchen porter.

Case history 8.2 – continued

The kitchen porter initially returned to work for 3 hours on 2 days a week during a quiet work period. He was specifically not allowed to lift any kitchen equipment or push trolleys but, with these caveats, he was allowed to undertake tasks on his job description which he felt capable of performing. In practical terms he operated the dishwashers, washed up manually and prepared vegetables with one of his colleagues doing any necessary lifting. He was made to feel welcome and, at his first assessment by the occupational physician after 2 weeks, he asked to increase his working hours. It was left to his discretion and that of his manager to implement the scheme outlined in Table 8.3 and with the task restrictions still in place. Assessment one month later revealed that he was working full time with restricted duties and, other than minor stump irritation, had had no problems.

He asked to extend his range of tasks and he graduated to loading food trolleys with individual meals and delivering the trolleys to wards nearest the kitchen. This distance was then extended. By 4 months he was working as a normal member of staff, fully integrated into the workplace. Subsequently there was no unexpected increase in injuries at work or sickness absence.

Anxiety and apprehension are important factors which may delay return to work after a lengthy period of absence even though the patient has regained full physical and mental capabilities. The underlying cause is a lack of confidence and the worry that basic skills may have been forgotten. Structured rehabilitation programmes with a gradual increase in the range of duties, hours worked, and resumption of responsibilities are of great benefit in overcoming these concerns. This case, which has been serialised to demonstrate various aspects of rehabilitation, is summarised in Fig. 8.2 to show the extent of a rehabilitation programme in its widest sense.

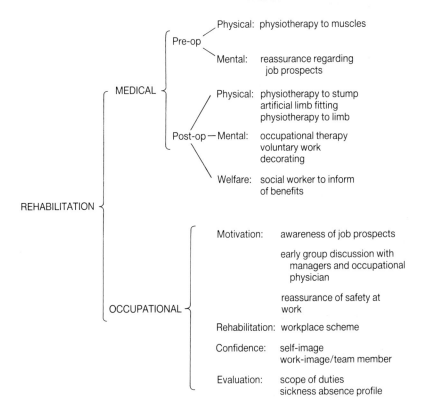

Fig. 8.2 Summary of the rehabilitation process

One further rehabilitation option is that of 'therapeutic' work. The patient is allowed to undertake limited work under 'medical' supervision as part of a hospital in or out-patient treatment programme while still meeting the basic definition of incapacity, which was stated in Chapter 7, to qualify for statutory sick pay or invalidity benefit. An example would be participation in light work to help recovery from psychiatric illness.

Case history 8.13

A 35 year-old records clerk developed acute anxiety and agoraphobia following the death of her mother. She was treated appropriately by her general practitioner with medication and regular counselling with the community psychologist. After 3 months of therapy the psychologist felt it would be helpful for her to resume limited part time working. She was referred to the occupational physician by her manager who was doubtful that this was a good idea as much of her work required meeting deadlines and dealing with members of the public.

At assessment she felt that she could manage 'a few hours a day in a quiet office where I don't have to meet people or answer the telephone!' Although she still had agoraphobia in the form of not liking crowded situations and being unable to travel on public transport, she had arranged that a friend would be able to provide transport to and from work. The manager was in fact very accommodating and created a job meeting the patient's requirements. Initially, she worked 2 mornings a week with gradual extension of the hours over a period of 2 months until she had resumed her normal commitments in terms of time. However, it was a further 2 months before she could resume the full extent of her job description.

Under the British benefits system, a formal programme must be agreed in advance with the Department of Social Security and earnings must be less than £35 per week. Therefore, at some stage during the scheme, a decision has to be made to terminate 'therapeutic' work, stop claiming benefit and resume normal payment from the employer. However, in times of economic stringency there are fewer opportunities for light work with the result that implementation of an occupational rehabilitation programme may have to be delayed until the patient is capable of undertaking normal duties for a limited time.

The importance of occupational rehabilitation is recognised in other countries. In the United States, where employers are obliged to bear directly more of the total cost of any illness or injury in their employees, the cost effectiveness of rehabilitation services in promoting independence and early return to work with sustained economic productivity is acknowledged. Experienced employees are seen to represent an investment, an appreciating asset and a resource to the firm. Retention must be set against the financial implications of recruitment and training new workers. The implementation of what is referred to as a 'recovery track programme' allows convalescents from service-related injuries to take temporary light duty jobs in which the employee works at an activity level compatible with his medical rehabilitation.

The programme commences with a counsellor being notified when an injured employee loses work time. This counsellor will continue to work with the employee until the maximum medical recovery is achieved and will also participate in both hospital and domiciliary visiting. On approval from the 'doctor providing clinical care' the employee enters the rehabilitation programme and is assessed every 30 days until maximum functioning is achieved or normal duties can be resumed. The employee is then followed up for a further 90 days in the normal work environment.

Following initial assessment or a periodic assessment of progress during the rehabilitation programme, it may be obvious that the employee will not be able to resume the previous work. The options to be considered in this situation are shown in Fig. 8.1 and include relocation within the same organisation following retraining either 'in house' or using one of the specialist agencies described below or, ultimately, retirement on health grounds.

Specialist rehabilitation services

Statutory provision of specific training and employment rehabilitation services began, in Britain, in the early 1900s when workshops and retraining centres were developed for disabled soldiers returning from the Boer and 1914-18 wars. Later, blind civilians were included in the schemes. Other disabled civilians were ineligible until during the Second World War. This widening of accessibility was created by the shortage of labour in industry and the need to maximise the potential for work of all civilians.

Until April 1991 the cornerstone of the current system was the Disablement Resettlement Officer (DRO), a civil servant employed as one of the Jobcentre team working under the auspices of the Department of the Employment. However, the organisation of services for people with disabilities has been changed in order to provide a more co-ordinated, flexible and local service for clients. The implementation of these changes occurred during 1992 with the creation of PACTs – integated Placing, Assessment and Counselling Teams whose members are known as Disability Employment Advisers (DEAs). They undertake the work previously performed by DROs, members of the Disablement Advisory Service (DAS) and Employment Rehabilitation Service (ERS) assessment teams.

One of their remits (the others are described in the section on the employment of the disabled (page 199) is to place job seekers with disabilities who require specialist occupational counselling and advice. To enable practical assessment of clients' abilities to be made, medical advice is obtained, in confidence, from the Department of Social Security's Regional Medical Services, individual hospital consultants, occupational physicians, Health and Safety Executive employment medical advisers and general practitioners. On receipt of the information, the client may be referred for assessment and retraining at an Employment Rehabilitation Centre (ERC) or skill centre, or may be advised to apply for jobs on the open market which are compatible with the disability. The job seeker may be advised to apply for further education courses such as business management or book keeping which will enable the acquisition of skills necessary to become self-employed, thus capitalising on knowledge and experience of a particular trade. Alternatively, the client may be advised to register as disabled. This is fully discussed later in this chapter.

The employment rehabilitation service operates 27 ERCs in the United Kingdom, two of which are residential. The aims are to

- re-establish a pattern of regular hours of work and rebuild confidence and morale.
- assess individual fitness for future employment or, if appropriate, vocational training.

The ERC has three functions, assessment, employment rehabilitation and job search training.

Assessment

This is undertaken by a team comprising the resettlement officer, employment medical adviser, social worker, ERC nursing sister, occupational psychologist, rehabilitation instructional officers and, in some centres, a remedial gymnast. The extent of the patient's disability and associated restrictions are assessed, psychometric testing is undertaken and the instructional officer assesses the aptitude of the patient in the various work options available, examples of which are described below. This process takes about 2 weeks following which a case conference is held and the patient then commences a rehabilitation programme.

Employment rehabilitation

The options include bench engineering, machine operating, woodwork, light assembly, for example, electrical and electronics, light packing, clerical/office, technology/book keeping and general activities such as labouring and gardening. The patient is placed in the most appropriate work section and, in general, this will last for 6 to 8 weeks. The maximum length of a placement is 6 months. Occasionally, after assessment, the patient may enter a work placement scheme with an external employer.

Job seeking skills

These are taught towards the end of and following the workplace scheme. The patient is taught how to prepare a curriculum vitae which maximises assets and abilities. Role play may be used to provide familiarisation with interview situations.

Referral to the ERC is not only the prerogative of the DEA. Patients can be referred by their hospital consultant, occupational physician or general practitioner or may refer themselves. While attending the centre the patient receives a tax free allowance which is larger than sickness or unemployment benefit, meals and lodging if required. There is also provision for a patient to attend, on a part time basis, while still requiring hospital treatment such as physiotherapy and receiving sickness benefit.

Having completed the course at the ERC there may be the need for further training in a particular skill in a more representative work environment. The patient can be referred from the ERC to a 'skill centre' or be referred directly by the DEA. The course will last 6 to 12 months with a similar range of options to those provided within the ERC. However, these courses are open to both the able bodied and the disabled. Skill centres became privatised and self-financing in 1990, since when there have been increasingly fewer places made available to those with disability who may have lower work rates and therefore be unable to meet production targets.

One of the most difficult problems following assessment is to decide who is likely to benefit most from early referral to either an 'in house' or a statutory rehabilitation scheme. Analysis of the return to work experiences of insurance claimants of working age and in employment at the time of injury at work or involvement in road traffic accidents has shown that severely injured accident victims are twice as likely to return to work as patients with progressive illness or serious acute illness. However, poor outcome, defined as a return to work rate of 20% or less, is associated with certain conditions such as back or spinal cord injury or psychological problems associated with severe head injury.

Ill-health retirement

To be told by an occupational physician, general practitioner or hospital consultant that consideration should be given to retiring on health grounds can be one of the most depressing, morale-sapping statements that a patient hears, even if it has been anticipated. The subject should not be raised until it becomes overwhelmingly clear that either the patient's health will preclude a return to the previous employment, for example, persistent exertional dyspnoea after myocardial infarction, or that the work environment will continue to adversely affect the patient's condition, for example occupational asthma when there are no opportunities for redeployment within the organisation. However, having made the recommendation, it is very important for the doctor to maintain a positive attitude and, having decided what the patient cannot do, begin to concentrate on what can be achieved and what skills there are to offer which may not only be workrelated but have developed in connection with hobbies and leisure activities. The patient must be aware of the facilities and scope of the services offered by the statutory agencies and how to access the system.

Case history 8.14

A 45 year-old painter developed pain in his cervical spine which was referred to both arms and associated with intermittent parasthesiae and numbness in the left arm, in the C6/7/8/T1 distributions. These symptoms were elicited during an annual health assessment which was undertaken as part of a voluntary health surveillance scheme for members of the works department. The painter had not complained voluntarily as he was afraid of losing his job.

Examination by the occupational physician revealed pain in the cervical spine with disability manifest by limitation of movement, weakness of the extensors of the forearm together with decreased grip strength. Impairment was confirmed by radiographs of the cervical spine which showed the presence of degenerative disc disease. He was referred for physiotherapy with resulting improvement in his symptoms and resolution of his neurological signs.

Six months later his symptoms returned. He requested to see the occupational physician who, on questioning the painter, also elicited a history of dizziness which was clearly associated with rotation and extension of his cervical spine. This had developed in the interim period. He did not want a further period of sickness absence. With the cooperation of his managers it was agreed that his work would be restricted in that he was not allowed to paint ceilings or high walls and, in addition, he would be allowed time to attend for physiotherapy. However, on this occasion, the severity and frequency of his symptoms progressed and he accepted that sickness absence was inevitable. Further Xrays showed progression of his degenerative disc disease and subluxation of the vertebral body of C6 on C7. He was referred for specialist advice.

After several lengthy discussions with the neurologist, neuro-surgeon and occupational physician, he decided to agree to cervical fusion knowing there was no guarantee that it would enable him to return to work as a painter. Assessment, 6 months following surgery, showed partial success in that he was pain free and had no neurological deficits. However, he lacked the cervical mobility that was necessary to enable him to fulfil his job description. There were no opportunities for relocation in the organisation.

He was referred, by the occupational physician and with the general practitioner's agreement, to the DRO while the papers were being processed for his retirement on health grounds. The DRO advised him that the best use of his skills would be to set up a small business. He was placed on specific courses to teach him the necessary practical management skills. Six months following his retirement he contacted the occupational physician to say that he was self-employed, having started a business as a painter and decorator, and had employed a young lad to undertake the physical aspects of the work which were outwith his own capabilities.

During the often lengthy assessment process it is important that morale and confidence are maintained. This can be achieved by suggesting participation in voluntary work which will not adversely affect benefit entitlement.

Case history 8.15

A 45 year-old firefighter was retired on medical grounds with chronic lumbar back pain consequent on degenerative disc disease. He had associated depression being very despondent and feeling that he was 'on the scrap heap'. Talking to him revealed that his hobby was birdwatching. He found that this was compatible with his back condition and provided him with relaxation and temporary abatement of his depression. He was encouraged to approach the warden of the nearby nature reserve to see if they could use his knowledge and interest as a voluntary warden with the freedom to come and go as he pleased depending on his mood. The warden was delighted to have extra help; the ex-firefighter became increasingly involved and his depression resolved; he was eventually appointed, when a vacancy arose, as a full-time employee.

Employment of the disabled

A proportion of men and women of working age will suffer an impairment resulting from an illness, accident or injury whether or not occupationally related and in spite of appropriate treatment and rehabilitation some of them will be left with a disability which may handicap them in terms of employability. Other men and women of working age will be handicapped as the result of congenital defects or illness, accident or injury during childhood. While managers often equate disability with poor work performance and an unsatisfactory attendance pattern, there is little objective evidence that disabled persons have above average sickness rates. Many show a strong motivation to overcome their disability and attendance rates are frequently better than average. Disability does not equate with ill health.

When medical fitness for work is assessed, it is the degree of any associated loss of function and any resulting disability or handicap which is important, matching, as one would for an able-bodied applicant, the balance between the patient's condition which should be interpreted in functional terms and the context of the job requirement. There is no evidence that disabled persons pose an increased safety risk either to themselves or to other employees when working in placements that are compatible with their capabilities. Communication and group meetings with the employee, line manager, personnel manager and occupational health staff are essential to identify placement needs. Any restrictions should be precisely stated and based on firm foundations.

The occupational physician should, if relevant, be able to give an opinion on the likelihood of progression of the disability and the potential need for special equipment and, or, modification of the working environment in the future to enable the job applicant to remain in employment for as long as is reasonably practical. This applies particularly to those who may have progressive impairment resulting in locomotor disabilities.

Case history 8.16

A 27 year-old lady applied to work as a senior training officer. The job involved formulating and writing management training policies, classroom teaching and assessing trainees in the workplace. She disclosed at her pre-employment health assessment that she suffered from motor-neurone disease. Her consent was obtained to ask for a report from her specialist in which questions were asked regarding the diagnosis, her current state of health and how the disease might progress in the future. At the time of her health interview she was noted to have an ataxic gait with weakness of her upper and lower limbs and slurred speech. She had difficulty with handwriting and in moving equipment. Mental function was unaffected.

Following the health assessment permission was given for the occupational physician to write to the employer outlining her current state of health, the effect that that might have on her performance and the fact that no unequivocal indication could be given as to the rate of progress of her disabilities other than that her condition would steadily deteriorate. The difficulties that this deterioration would cause in oral communication were stressed. The Director of Personnel sanctioned her employment.

This case history is continued on page 203 to illustrate the use of services available to enable disabled persons to remain in work.

Statistics

The Office of Populations Censuses and Surveys (OPCS) published a 'Survey of Disability in Great Britain in 1989'. Report No.4 showed that of people under pensionable age assessed as having difficulties with daily activities only 31% were employed at the time of the survey. With reference to the categories of personal disability which are listed in Table 8.1, a survey of the prevalence of disabilities in the population as a whole showed that locomotor problems are the most common affecting more than 4 million adults. This represents an overall prevalence rate of 99 per 1000 of the population aged 16–74 years. In this category arthritis is a major contribuent. This category is followed by hearing (prevalence rate 59 per 1000 population) and problems associated with personal care (prevalence rate 57 per 1000 of the population). These statistics are illustrated in Fig. 8.3.

As might be expected the prevalence rises sharply with age as shown in Fig. 8.4.

Legislation

The recruitment of disabled civilians, in Britain, to ease the labour shortage during World War II led to the passing of the Disabled Persons (Employment)

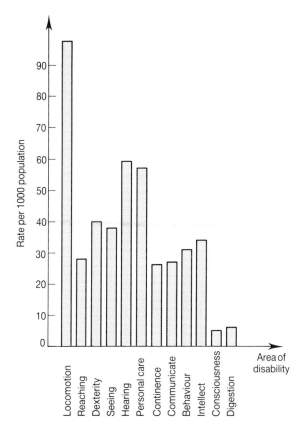

Fig. 8.3 Prevalence of disability in the adult population (> 16 years) in Great Britain by type of disability

Act in 1944 which was later amended in 1958. For the purpose of the Act a disabled person is defined as:

> a person with a disability which substantially handicaps him in obtaining or keeping employment or in undertaking work on his own account of a kind which, apart from the disability, would normally be suited to the age, qualification or experience of that person.

The disability must be likely to last for at least 12 months.
The provisions of the Act are:

- to establish a register of disabled people for employment.
- to establish a framework for the provision of vocational rehabilitation training and resettlement services for disabled people.
- to establish a quota system for employers to promote the employment of

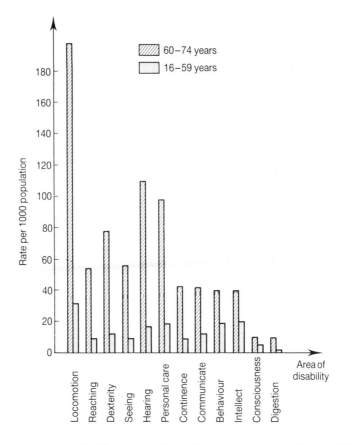

Fig. 8.4   Prevalence of disability in the adult population in Great Britain by type of disability and age

registered disabled people. Any firm with 20 or more employees should have among them at least 3% with a registered disability.
- to provide sheltered employment.
- to establish a National Advisory Council and Local Disablement Advisory Committees as sources of advice in respect of the employment and training of disabled people.

Financial and advisory services for disabled people

The services are administered by the Department of Employment and not the National Health Service. Therefore formal referral is needed between the two systems. The overall lack of awareness of the facilities available by general medical practitioners has resulted in both lack of referral and inappropriate referrals. Integration of specialists previously known by individual titles, such as the Disablement Resettlement Officer, the Blind Person's Resettlement Officer, Hospital Resettlement Officers (who are few in number) and members of the Disablement Advisory Service, into PACTs will lead to a coordinated service. Members of each regional team are available to advise employers on the aids and services available to facilitate the initial or continuing employment of disabled persons; such services are:

- cash grants to make adaptations to premises or to provide equipment, for example, building ramps or installing special toilet facilities. They are available for any disabled person.
- free provision of special aids to employment on a permanent basis for individual registered disabled persons. Examples are electrical tricycles, voice operated computers and visual aids such as closed circuit television systems. Voice operated computers enable the severely disabled person to do anything which is normally processed through a keyboard. Voice commands can now control robot arms on assembly lines thus opening up opportunities for the employment of the disabled in the office, on the shop floor and at home.
- financial assistance for registered disabled persons to get to work, for example, the cost of taxi fares.
- job introduction schemes available to all disabled persons and accessed by the DEA.
- personal reader schemes for the visually handicapped.

The scope of these schemes can be illustrated by the story of the lady with motor neurone disease.

Case history 8.16 (continued)

Within 3 years of commencing work as a training officer, her motor-neurone disease had progressed. The occupational physician received a letter from the training manager asking for advice to enable them to cope with the deterioration which had taken place since her appointment. They asked in particular for advice on 'mobility, using computer keyboard, car adaptations and appropriate support groups'. At that time the training officer had difficulty in using a typewriter and keyboard owing to increasing weakness and ataxia. She required aids to use the toilets and lunch was brought to her desk. Subsequently she became unable to use the telephone and ultimately to drive her modified car. At each stage in the progression of the disease a meeting was held with the employee, her manager, the occupational physician and the occupational health nurse.

The first step was to provide a wheelchair at work and volunteers were recruited (from among her colleagues) to help her from her car morning and night to the wheelchair and take her to the office, to take her to the toilet facilities which were adapted for disabled usage and to provide help in the event of fire. As her disability progressed, the occupational health sister approached the following agencies for advice; Local Authority Social Worker, Association of Independent Disabled Selfsufficiency (AIDS), the Disablement Information Advice Line (DIAL), Disability Alliance, the Royal Association for Disability and Rehabilitation (RADAR) and DAS. A voice operated computer was provided by the DAS and she also changed to part-time working totalling eighteen and a half hours per week. When she became more severely handicapped, she employed a 'helper' who took over the former voluntary roles of her colleagues. Using these various services her employment was able to be significantly extended.

Case history 8.17

A consultant radiologist developed multiple sclerosis at the age of 35 years shortly after his appointment. The disease followed a slowly progressive course until, 20 years following onset, he was having difficulty, due to weakness, in walking round the hospital site, attending ward rounds and lectures. His balance was impaired and he was restricted in the extent of patient screening which could be safely undertaken. The physical fatigue also affected mental functioning particularly in terms of concentration. After much persuasion by the occupational health sister he agreed to investigate the use of a wheelchair. This was provided by the DAS and had a limited benefit in increasing his range of mobility and, thereby, lessening his mental fatigue. Subsequent technical developments made available an electric tricycle which was again provided by the DAS (Fig. 8.5). This greatly extended his range of mobility allowing him

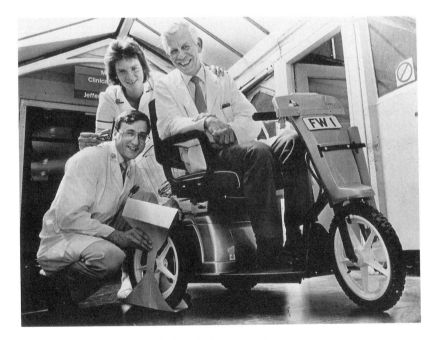

Fig. 8.5   Mobility in Action

to attend ward rounds, clinical meetings and lectures, conserved his physical strength and thereby lessened mental fatigue and its associated effects. He was affectionately provided with his own, personalised number plates FW 1 by members of his department.

Disabled persons register

Keeping the register of disabled people for employment is yet another role of the DEA. It is a voluntary register, set up under the 1944 Act, to help the disabled gain employment. Medical evidence may be required in support of the application to the effect that there is a disability which is likely to cause a substantial impairment of the individual's prospects of obtaining or retaining employment. The certificate of registration "green card" is valid for a minimum of one year and a maximum of 10 years.

There are advantages and disadvantages to registration. The advantages are the potential for preferential treatment under the quota system and the availability of 'designated' employment, e.g. passenger electric lift attendants and car park attendants. However, as car park attendants are increasingly expected to undertake security duties, the opportunities for employment of the disabled in this area are diminishing. Further advantages are immediate entitlement to certain social security benefits and services and the opportunity for employment in sheltered workshops for those with very severe physical or mental handicaps.

What are the disadvantages? Frequently there is self-perception of social stigma and there is the disadvantage in the job market for those with relatively minor handicaps due to the employer's misconceptions of the description 'disabled'. The register does not take account of the nature of the disability so that someone who is severely handicapped registers in the same way as someone who may only have a minor impairment. This allows employers to reach their 'quota' of disabled persons without necessarily employing people with severe disability. Within the population of working age there are probably at least as many unregistered as registered disabled persons. The facilities of government agencies are available to registered and non-registered disabled persons alike.

Quota

As already stated, employers of 20 or more persons must employ 3% of registered disabled persons. In 1987 25% of employers in this group fulfilled this obligation. The compliance in 1991 is even less.

Sheltered employment

This is available to those who are so severely disabled, as judged by the DEA, to be unlikely to obtain or keep a job in 'open' employment. The options include factories, sheltered workshops and sheltered placement schemes organised by Remploy, Local Authorities and Voluntary Agencies such as the Spastics Society and RADAR. MENCAP, a charitable organisation catering for the needs of those who are mentally handicapped and their families, operates a pathway employment service which is a job introduction scheme. In 1985 there were 127 workshops run by local authorities and voluntary bodies and 89 factories organised by Remploy. Many 'users' have psychiatric disabilities, mental handicap or severe physical handicap as a result of, for example, spina bifida, cerebral palsy or epilepsy.

Future prospects

In 1989 the Health and Safety Executive published Guidance Note MS23 'Health aspects of job placement and rehabilitation advice to employers' which advised employers to ask the question, 'can the person do the job in question regardless of any physical or mental health problems? In February 1992 there was an attempt to introduce new legislation, 'The Civil Rights (Disabled Persons) Bill', which made it illegal for anyone to use disability as a reason for withholding equal treatment whether in housing, employment, education, transport, leisure or any other public or private services. Unfortunately it failed to gain a second reading and has, for the time being, been abandoned. Nevertheless, with increasing awareness, knowledge of and use of the facilities and services available to facilitate the employment of disabled people, more opportunities are being created.

Benefits

In Chapter 7 an outline was given of the range of benefits relative to ill-health in Britain. Sickness and invalidity benefit were discussed in detail in relation to long-term sickness absence. However, two non-contributory benefits,

- disability living allowance (DLA)
- severe disablement allowance (SDA)

are available for those who, following rehabilitation, remain significantly handicapped. The disability living allowance was introduced in April 1992 replacing the attendance allowance and mobility allowance which were amended and subsumed into the new arrangements. A 'means tested' benefit

- disability working allowance (DWA)

was also introduced in April 1992. In addition, consideration must be given to the part that benefits can play in creating incentives or disincentives to return to work after illness or injury. As with other benefits that require application, for example industrial injury benefit, people will not apply for them unless they are aware of their existence and their own entitlement. Doctors in all specialties play a large part in increasing that awareness and therefore the new benefits will be described in some detail.

In social security terms, impairment is translated into the concept of loss of faculty which may be defined as 'any pathological condition or any loss or reduction of the normal physical or mental function of some organ or part of the body including disfigurement'. Disability is regarded as the inability, which arises from the loss of faculty, to do things or to do them as well as a person of the same age and sex whose physical and mental condition is normal. Disablement is the overall effect of the relevant disabilities, that is, the overall inability to perform the normal activities of life and the loss of health, strength and power to enjoy a normal life.

Disability living allowance

This was introduced in April 1992 as a non-contributory benefit to extend and replace the attendance allowance (for people disabled before the age of 65 years) and the mobility allowance. Attendance allowance will continue for people whose care needs first arise after the age of 65 years. The DLA is non-contributory, not means tested, not taxed and entitles patients to increased levels of income support, housing and community charge benefit. The new arrangements introduce new lower rates of benefits for some less disabled people not currently entitled to benefits. The DLA has two components, mobility and care. Qualifying factors are:

- The claimant must be incapable of work by reason of some specific disease or bodily or mental disablement. Legally, claimants have to prove on the balance of probabilities that there is no work which they can reasonably be expected to do, taking into account their age, education, experience, state of health and other personal factors. 'Work' is defined as part-time or full-time work for which an employer would be prepared to pay or self-employed work in some gainful occupation.
- The claimant must be resident in the UK and have been domiciled in the UK for the previous 26 weeks.
- The claimant must have been unwell for the past 3 months. The cause of the condition does not need to be definitely defined, the main criterion being the effect on the patient. For those who are terminally ill the qualifying time is waived.
- To qualify for the mobility component the claimant must be between the ages of 5 and 65 years; for the care component the age range is 16–65 years.

The mobility component of the DLA is paid at two rates. The higher rate corresponds to the pre-existing rules for mobility allowance which are:

- complete inability to walk
- virtual inability to walk
- exertion would be dangerous to present state of health
- deafness
- blindness
- loss of both feet (amputee)
- severe mental impairment with severe behavioural problems.

To qualify for the higher rate the incapacity to walk must be due to physical disablement and not mental impairment, for example, agoraphobia or personality disorders. While the use of artificial aids such as artificial limbs and crutches is taken into account, factors such as stairs, hills, distance to shops or work, are not. The manner of walking, for example, stumbling or swaying may be relevant but discomfort, for example, walking although in severe pain, is disregarded. Although the award of the allowance is related to the ability to walk outside, the assessment usually takes place indoors leading to false conclusions being made. The claim must take into account all available evidence and therefore the claimant must present the worst possible case and not make light of the functional effects of the disability.

The lower rate is paid to those who can walk but require help and, or, guidance if in unfamiliar surroundings. This might apply to persons with dementia, those who are visually impaired and those with learning difficulties. The mobility component of the DLA can continue for life and is payable if the applicant is in hospital, residential care or an institution.

The care component of the DLA is payable at one of three rates as summarised in Table 8.4.

Table 8.4 Differential rates of care components of the disability living allowance

Highest rate	– those who are terminally ill
	– those who require attention*, i.e. services of an active nature, or supervision*, i.e. services which may be anticipatory and precautionary, day and night
Middle rate	– those who require attention or supervision day or night
	– those requiring home dialysis automatically qualify for this rate, those treated with continuous ambulatory peritoneal dialysis do not
Lowest rate	– those who require help with bodily functions for part of the day
	– those who do not pass the cooking test*

Note: * see text for explanation

Attention refers to reasonably requiring attention from another person in connection with bodily functions which persons would normally do for themselves. For payment at the lowest rate attention is required for a significant portion of the day for at least 4 days per week. At the middle and higher rates attention is required frequently throughout the day; prolonged (20 minutes) or repeated (at least twice) throughout the night; both day and night for at least 4 days per week.

Supervision in the daytime is defined as continual supervision from another person throughout the day in order to avoid substantial damage to the individual or another. At night time supervision refers to the need for another person to be awake for a prolonged period or at frequent intervals to watch over the individual in order to avoid substantial damage to the individual or others.

The Cooking Test describes the ability to prepare a 'cooked main meal' if provided with the ingredients. It assesses the client's ability to lift, turn taps, plan a meal and safely work in a kitchen. It does not assess the ability to shop for the ingredients nor does it take into account the availability of ready cooked meals. Do you think that the provision of a microwave cooker and fridge/freezer would disbar the disabled person from claiming this lower rate of the care component?

The decision to award DLA is based on perception of need rather than on what is actually provided. Loss of function is the overriding criterion and applicants with asthma, heart disease, arthritis, multiple sclerosis and senile dementia have been successful. A disabled person living alone can still qualify for the allowance.

The method of application for the DLA has been revised. The new arrangements for assessment and adjudication are based on a form completed by the applicant. Medical examination is no longer essential. A relevant person, whether doctor, nurse, occupational therapist or 'someone like this' is required to enter details of the diagnosis but is not expected to read or confirm the applicant's statement nor undertake any medical examination. An appeal system has been incorporated to a Tribunal consisting of a lawyer, general practitioner and 'caring person' who will discuss the disputed issues with the applicant.

Disability working allowance

This was introduced in April 1992 as an income-related benefit for people with disabilities which limit their ability to compete for jobs but who want to work. It can be claimed as well as DLA but it is means-tested and may reduce the amount of housing and community charge benefits.

Claimants must be over 16 with an illness or disability which puts them at a disadvantage in getting a job; they must be in receipt of benefits listed in Table 8.5; and they must be in paid employment for at least 16 hours per week including self-employment

Assets taken into account when accessing the amount include income, some social security benefits, and savings between certain limits. They exclude

Table 8.5   Receipt of benefits permitting entitlement to the disability working allowance

---

Invalidity Benefit *or*
Severe Disablement Allowance *or*
Disability premium *with*
      Income support   for at least 1/56
      Housing Benefit   days before claim
      Community Charge Benefit

                                  OR

Disability Living Allowance *or*
Industrial Injuries Disablement Benefit *or*
War Disablement Pension

                                  OR

Invalid 3 wheeler from DSS

DLA. The award of family credit and DWA are mutually exclusive. Ironically, the person most likely to benefit will be single, living at home with parents and with no dependents. Other potential claimants may find that the restrictions outweigh their entitlements to other benefits and that they could therefore end up financially disadvantaged.

Severe disability allowance

This benefit was introduced in 1983. It is non-contributory and available for persons under the age of 65 years who

- are 80% disabled
- have been unable to work continuously for 28 weeks
- have lived in Great Britain for at least 10 out of the previous 20 years
- have been present in Great Britain for 24 out of the previous 28 weeks.

The system is based on the concept of traumatic loss. However it does not deal adequately with either physical or mental chronic ill health. Automatic qualification is assured by the receipt of DLA and assessment as 80% disabled based on the scale of disability under the industrial injuries scheme (see Chapter 4). The receipt of vaccine damage payments and registration as blind or partially sighted are other automatic qualifying factors. The allowance has, theoretically, a wide catchment population. For example, it is applicable to married women and those disabled from childhood who meet the residential qualifications but have never actually worked. The difficulty is to prove 80% disablement unless one of the automatic qualifying factors has been met. Receipt of the SDA provides eligibility to the disability premium linked with income support, housing and community charge benefit. Adverse factors are that it may be difficult for sufferers of chronic physical or psychiatric conditions to substantiate a claim. It also discriminates against ethnic minorities who may have lived abroad.

9

Health promotion in the workplace

Summary

Health promotion in the workplace must start with the correct assessment of the risks to health arising from work, communication of information about them and appropriate control measures. Thus health promoting activities should be part of an integral strategy that controls the highest work-related risks as well as addressing other means of maintaining health and well being. They should also arise opportunistically out of many individual contacts with workers. In the development of important strategies regarding smoking, alcohol and other substance abuse there must be consultation, education, individual counselling and other support as well as an explicit policy. Lasting and wide ranging improvement in reducing psychological stress is more likely following the identification and remedy of organisational causes of stress than merely by focussing on individual behaviour. Immunisation should address work-related risks in the first instance. Influencing dietary habits, and encouraging weight reduction and exercise are laudable aims, especially if in tandem with health protection measures. Inappropriate 'screening' does not promote health and may foster unwarranted anxiety. It is no substitute for the good practice of preventive occupational medicine.

Introduction to promotion of good health

The purpose of this chapter is to consider practical aspects of the promotion of health among the working population. It takes into account the special opportunities and difficulties associated with workplace health promotion and complements Chapter 5 in particular. Promoting health in the workplace is part of the U.K. Government's policy statement: 'The Health of the Nation' and is an important feature of the policy of many other national Governments and International bodies such as the European Community and the World Health Organisation. This last mentioned organisation has defined health as a state of complete physical, mental and social well being and not merely the absence of disease or infirmity. Health promotion at work can mean different priorities to different people (Fig. 9.1). The following account utilises practical illustrations of the common issues.

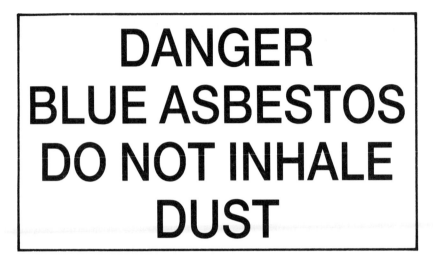

Fig. 9.1 This sign was affixed to the door of a hospital boilerhouse (just across the carpark from the chest clinic). Clearly the hospital authorities were naively assuming that they were educating their workers on health hazards at work. Presumably, as far as they were concerned, it was then up to the employees to reduce their risks by doing their utmost not to breathe at work!

Health promotion in the workplace should aim to:

- educate employees and employers in the risks to health arising from work and other factors
- Influence the attitudes and hence the behaviour of employees and employers in relation to the promotion of their health and the health of others.
- Provide facilities and assistance to fulfil the above aims.

Case history 9.1

A firm manufacturing fine tools embarked on, and publicised, a health promotion exercise. This included offering a wide range of high fibre, low fat meals in the staff canteen, providing exercise facilities, and classes to help in stopping smoking. Many executives and a proportion of other staff but not many manual workers took advantage of this. Many employees still brought in their own lunches or went out for chips and beer at lunch time. Few employees who did not previously engage in physical exercise, started to do so as a result of this programme.

In the meantime, some employees in parts of the firm continued to suffer from occupational diseases of the skin, lungs and of hearing as evident during their attendances at the Occupational Health Department or when referred by their general practitioner to hospital outpatient specialists. A clear strategy and mechanism for preventing many of these cases or managing their consequences was lacking.

Clearly, before beginning to assess priorities for preventive medicine in a workplace certain important considerations need to be understood; the failure of preventive action can often be traced back to neglect of one or more of these factors listed here.

A workforce is not a random sample of the community from which it is derived

Quite apart from obvious differences in age and gender from the general population there may be important differences in health and in attitudes to health and safety. Thus because of various selection processes on appointment and during employment, employees may be healthier as a group than age and gender matched counterparts from the same social and geographical background. Employment is also associated with a selection process based on social, cultural and educational background. Thus salaried white collar employment would generally be more likely than waged blue collar employment to favour recruiting employees with healthier prospects. Jobs with high risk such as construction, especially if without security of tenure, might be more likely to attract employees willing to accept higher risks to their health and safety and this culture might be reinforced by peer pressure within the workplace.

Employees within a particular workplace are not a 'captive audience'.

All employees are expected to fulfil the terms of their contract of employment and since most of them do this to various degrees their activities at work will follow similar patterns. However beyond this, the extent to which each will participate in health promotion is influenced by many complex factors which are outlined or illustrated later. A simplistic attitude on the part of well-intentioned health promoters might not be needed for those in the workplace who are already motivated in pursuing a healthy lifestyle and at the same time might exert no influence on the others who remain indifferent.

Work itself may include very important determinants of health

The risks to health from work needed to be systematically addressed as described earlier (Chapter 5). There are various reasons for this: the legal and moral responsibility of the employer is to reduce occupational risks to health and not those pertaining to the community as a whole. Occupational risks to health may be substantial, but at the same time very remediable in terms of cost effectiveness. Employees who perceive that the conditions of their job exert an important adverse influence on their health, safety or wellbeing are not likely to be responsive or sympathetic to health promotion attempts that explicitly or implicitly ignore these concerns. Sadly, all too often firms embark on screening programmes which bear no relation to the prevention of work related illhealth, and neglect simple and obvious means of assessing and controlling serious health risks from occupational hazards in their workplace. There are several reasons for this. Often there is ignorance of the important points outlined above. Sometimes, pursuing policies of 'health promotion' that bear no specific relation to the workplace in question can be a convenient path of least resistance for all concerned – employers, employees and occupational health departments. Thus for employers it presents an image of doing something while not opening any cans of worms; employees feel that something is being done for their health which would not have a bearing on their employment prospects; while occupational health departments may be pleased to find a health related issue which enjoys the support both of employers and employees. This can be particularly true in an adverse economic climate, since employers might avoid anything that could increase costs and reduce productivity and competitiveness. At the same time employees might be wary of occupational health activities which they might perceive as reducing job prospects for the workplace as a whole, or for individuals, in a climate of unemployment or of reducing overtime work. Thus a consenses commitment to some form of health promotion which is aimed at individual lifestyle rather than at workplace risks can appear an attractive soft option, and relatively risk-free or inexpensive compared to some of the measures described in Chapter 5, or to a pay rise!

Workers should be involved in health promotion

Health promotion exercises determined by senior policy makers and filtered down through the ranks, might not earn the support of an often suspicious workforce. Indeed patronising attempts to predicate from on high may alienate a proportion of the workers.

Case history 9.2

A well-intentioned manager in a large National Health Service hospital decided to introduce a programme of health promotion. A detailed policy was worked out, based on his concept of what the workforce needed, and included action on smoking, healthy eating, exercise and stress management. A committee was established to set the wheels in motion, including union representatives. Many members of the committee not only smoked but also considered themselves experts on stress management. The meetings of the committee, taking part against a background of management–union dispute with respect to NHS reorganisation and redundancies, became a stage for argument about provision of recreational facilities, time off work for counselling and places for smokers to smoke! The project came to an unsatisfactory end when the manager was himself declared redundant.

Workplace issues

Assessment of needs

As with most of the methods described in this book, a thorough assessment is a crucial first step before embarking on any intervention.

Case history 9.3

An employer in a large service organisation sought the advice of an occupational physician for the purpose of launching a healthy workplace strategy. The personnel officer tabled various suggestions including changing the balance of food available in the canteen together with appropriate labelling, weight reduction and 'stop smoking' classes, exercise facilities, mammography, cholesterol and cervical screening. The physician reviewed various sources of information and found that the employer was not fulfilling the legal quota for employing disabled employees, was doing very little if anything to rehabilitate its own employees when off sick, even when disabled by their work, and was tending to press for premature illhealth retirement in many cases. Health surveillance in relation to skin and respiratory hazards of occupation was scanty while a disproportionately large resource was devoted to initial health assessment of job applicants. Many employees and some managers were very ignorant of the health risks arising from their work or on the means of reducing these risks. First aid provision was less than that required by law. The physician pointed out the contradictions between the professed aim to promote health and the plethora of ideas to modify lifestyle on the one hand, and the many shortcomings that he had found in regarding health protection in relation to work. The outcome of his advice is unknown.

As this case history shows, before the physician endorsed what the personnel manager had planned, the information relevant to 'health at work' in that workplace was sought. What was found was not all encouraging and led to the conclusion that the employers probably had the wrong priorities. It may be very tempting for health professionals to address a single issue, or a set of health promotion related issues, in isolation when asked to do so. However they should exert their professional skills and judgement to view the whole picture and to give balanced advice on the basis of this.

Opportunistic health promotion

Opportunistic health promotion for the individual employee can be a very powerful instrument although reaching only a fraction of the workforce. Consider the following case:

Case history 9.4

An accounts clerk presented to the occupational physician complaining of sore feet and wondering whether he had 'athlete's foot'. The physician explained that such complaints would not normally be dealt with in the occupational health department but agreed to examine the feet on the understanding that further management would be undertaken by the general practitioner. The feet were slightly swollen and the webs between the toes macerated. The employee jokingly conceded that he had slept in his shoes and socks. Further enquiry and examination revealed a substantial alcohol intake (to the order of 5 units per day), heavy smoking, symptoms consistent with chronic bronchitis, poor dietary habits, unsatisfactory oral hygiene and slight overweight.

The physician enquired in detail about the patient's habits but in a nonjudgemental way and provided answers to the patient's questions that followed the detailed clinical assessment. The patient then asked for the physician's advice on diet, smoking and rational alcohol consumption. This was provided verbally, backed up by health education literature, target setting and a review appointment with the occupational health nurse. The general practitioner was consulted and agreed to this plan. Over a period of a few months the patient's alcohol consumption fell to about 14 units per week, his weight was restored to normal, he stopped smoking, and resumed attending the dentist. His feet improved with basic personal hygiene and without specific treatment.

While the above approach can only deal with a small proportion of a workforce it has a high chance of succeeding. The employee/patient has spontaneously asked for assessment and advice which is then objectively provided. The employee knows that the assessment need not be accepted nor the advice necessarily followed, but having presented with this in mind is more likely to follow it. The employee's attitude is positive from the start and likely to remain so provided a patronising attitude is not adopted and the option of self-determination remains. Such an attitude can slowly but surely permeate a workforce, as in the following case history.

Case history 9.5

A trained occupational physician was appointed in a part-time capacity for a chemical firm that had previously employed the services of a general practitioner. In the first few sessions many employees walked in quietly with their shirt sleeves rolled up waiting for their yearly blood test. The new physician then discovered that it had been the practice for production workers to have a yearly estimation of liver function tests and full blood count. On an initial site visit by the occupational physician mainly respiratory and cutaneous hazards were evident but none for which blood tests were routinely indicated as a form of health surveillance. The occupational physician engaged the workers individually in conversation, found out about their jobs, their lifestyles, their general state of health and their attitudes to it. Most employees welcomed the opportunity to sit down and be listened to. A minority of employees complained to their union representatives and hence to the factory manager that 'the new doctor had stopped the blood tests'. The physician explained the reasoning for abandoning the tests to the factory manager, conceded that further explanation may be needed, and asked for the opportunity of participating in safety committee meetings, where he explained the reasons for taking detailed occupational histories, and the limited value of blood tests in that particular context. This was paralleled by regular workplace visits by the physician.

The spontaneous consultation rate increased, concerns about health in relation to work or other factors were more openly addressed both within the confines of the clinic and of the safety committee which became better attended by safety representatives and senior managers. On average one new health related issue was placed on the agenda for each meeting and discussed following a short presentation by the physician. Discussion thereafter was generally fruitful, resulting in an agreed plan of action on both occupational health and lifestyle issues.

Health education is brought about by imparting knowledge, then changing attitudes and eventually changing behaviour. This can be achieved by two approaches: the more individual approach exemplified by case history 9.4, or the 'campaign' approach. Case history 9.5, shows the middle road between the former and the latter. It has a great deal to commend it especially in small- or medium-sized traditional workplaces. The size of these makes it easier than in a large organisation for a substantial proportion of the workforce to be met opportunistically and individually. Health education is best embarked upon in manageable groups or through a forum such as the safety committee with employee participation. Thus concerns experienced by workers as individuals or expressed collectively, are taken seriously, freely discussed and then progressed as part of an open health promotion strategy. Involvement with workers' representatives should be early and active and not merely an afterthought to help in 'carrying it through'.

Having discussed assessment of the need for health promotion and the different approaches to introducing this, the rest of the chapter will deal with individual issues not covered elsewhere in the text in more detail.

Nonsmoking policies

A large proportion of smokers are aware and accept that tobacco smoking can seriously harm their health. Many of them would like to stop if they had the opportunity to do so. The working community can be an important peer pressure group, and with the right culture and support it can help in reducing the prevalence of smoking (although if the culture favours smoking and there is inadequate alternative support, smoking habits are often fostered). Therefore the workplace can be a crucial setting for reducing the scourge of tobacco smoking. Furthermore, there is now good epidemiological evidence of the risks of exposure to sidestream tobacco smoke (passive smoking), and debate about this issue in terms of health and safety at work is leading employers increasingly towards nonsmoking policies.

Case history 9.6

A bus driver had been employed for several years by a company which allowed its passengers to smoke, long after the epidemiological evidence of the harmful effects of inhaling tobacco smoke was available. He had never smoked and yet he developed cancer of the bronchus. He sued his employer, arguing that his cancer was, more likely than not, caused by his passive inhalation of sidestream tobacco smoke at work. The case was settled out of court by the bus company paying a substantial sum to the driver.

This case history illustrates the dilemma faced by employers when faced by a vociferous group insisting on freedom to smoke and an equally forceful lobby demanding unpolluted air. The recent evidence, accepted increasingly by courts and tribunals that passive smoking may cause fatal disease now tips the balance firmly in favour of the introduction of non-smoking policies. How, therefore does one reduce tobacco smoking in the workplace. Consider the following example.

Case history 9.7

A health authority decided that it wished to set an example in relation to health promotion in the workplace. It decreed that as from a specific date, all smoking by staff was prohibited on its premises, and disciplinary proceedings (which could lead to dismissal) would be instituted against any staff member caught flouting the rule. A female domestic assistant who had smoked all her life found that all of a sudden she could not do so. Even most of her official breaks were not long enough for her to change into her outdoor clothing and go and smoke outside the premises. She resigned her job but promptly instituted proceedings alleging constructive dismissal.

What went wrong? Put yourself in the position of employees of different persuasions and analyse the situation. Clearly the smokers felt that they could not accept such a sudden imposition. They neither had the time to come to terms with it nor an alternative smoking zone for their breaks. However, what about the nonsmokers? They had not been made adequately aware of the risks of passive smoking and, except for the few who were appreciably upset by their colleagues smoking, were therefore not particularly concerned with, nor necessarily supportive of, the policy. Moreover some of the employees, especially those active in trade union spheres, felt that in this, as on any other issue directly affecting habits and practice in the workplace, the management should have consulted with the workforce. Lack of consultation was an 'infringement of workers' rights' no matter how apparently worthy the cause was. An organisation that wishes to promote health at work through the reduction or abolition of tobacco smoking in the workplace should therefore do the following:

- encourage and engage in debate on the issue, for example in safety committees.
- inform all concerned about the evidence of the risks associated with tobacco smoking
- agree with consensus between employers and employees, both a time schedule for implementation of the policy and its rules, and also the facilities to be provided to help employees give up smoking.
- provide and publicise appropriate stopping smoking groups and clinics, with a balance of professional support and self-help.
- provide clearly designated smoking areas for employees who wish to continue smoking, during their breaks, after implementation of the non-smoking rules.

Some firms may feel that the above is too complex or difficult to handle without the advice and support of external agencies. Help for firms that wish to implement non-smoking policies is available, notably from the charity ASH (Action on Smoking and Health).

Alcohol abuse

More so than tobacco smoking, misuse of alcohol or other substances can have implications with respect to work. Thus, it can harm the patient directly regardless of occupation, it can increase safety risks at work for the patient and workmates, and it leads to reduced performance and absenteeism at work. All firms should have a policy in relation to alcohol and other substance abuse and the physician should advise on it.

Case history 9.8

A 55 year-old supervisor was referred for the first time to the occupational physician because she had become intolerable to work with and was performing very poorly. Her manager said that her colleagues 'would no longer carry her' and they had got to 'the end of the line'. He requested that she be retired on the grounds of ill health or that her employment be terminated on the grounds of incapacity but as far as he and her workmates were concerned they were not ready to accept her back at work. The occupational physician made further enquiries and found that the worker's alcohol problem had been known, and had caused some difficulties at her work, for at least 5 years.

This was a case of too little and too late. The alcohol policy as well as providing for general education about the health risks of alcohol should make early intervention the rule. It should guarantee confidentiality for the victim and reassurance that so long as the policy and advice are followed, the firm will allow sickness absence for the problem to be dealt with. Earlier referral to the occupational health department could have permitted the worker to have recognised her problem and curtailed her alcohol consumption sooner, and her colleagues would not have been driven to the limit of their endurance.

The occupational physician said that the referral should have been made years previously and that the function of the occupational health service was to assist in rehabilitating workers with alcohol problems. The manager reluctantly agreed to accept the worker back at work after a period of sickness absence during which a rehabilitation and monitoring programme was agreed in conjunction with her and an alcohol counsellor. Unfortunately after her return to work in a supernumery and monitored capacity her alcohol abuse did not improve. Despite repeated warnings she continued to drink heavily mainly on her own, and was abusive to her colleagues and customers and she tried to deceive and manipulate both the physician and the counsellor. After a final disciplinary hearing she was dismissed.

Case history 9.9

A 47 year-old porter was formally referred to the occupational physician because of his alcohol problem. He had been noted to be late for work and hungover on some mornings, usually after payday or after a weekend off. Sometimes he came back late and smelling of alcohol after lunch breaks. His manager had given him a formal warning but said that he would support him provided he followed professional advice and showed reasonable goodwill and signs of improvement. The physician found that the worker lived alone, his only close relative being his mother, and socialised with a group of friends who drank heavily. He had no understanding of the relative alcohol content of various drinks and measures. Until the formal warning by his manager he had not realised how noticeably poor his performance had become, and he was particularly shaken by the prospect of losing his job. The physician reviewed the alcohol history in detail, at the same time taking the opportunity to explain the alcohol content of various drinks. The porter was given a diary in which to record his alcohol consumption every day and was reviewed at frequent intervals by the physician or nurse. During the counselling he acknowledged the role of peer pressure in fostering his drinking habits and followed the physician's advice to change his circle of friends. This took some time but was eventually achieved. About nine months after the original referral, the worker, his manager and the physician were in agreement that he no longer had an alcohol-related problem, that he was a valued member of the workforce and that no further follow-up was needed, although like other workers on that site he was aware of the availability of the occupational health service for advice and support at any time should he need it.

From the above case histories, it should be clear that in implementing an alcohol policy for the workplace, the following points should be considered:

- an explicit statement that alcohol abuse can and is a recognised problem in that workplace, but one which the employers and employees are committed to resolve
- information and education on the risks associated with alcohol abuse, on their recognition and on rational safe drinking practices
- clear rules on whether, where and when alcohol drinking at work (including breaks) is allowed, and summary disciplinary rules (e.g. about drink-driving)
- explicit routes and mechanisms including both self-referral and formal management referral of employees who may have an alcohol-related problem, for help by the occupational health department. This has to be accompanied by availability of leave of sickness absence, and of job security. These would continue to apply so long as the individual complied with the specialist advice given
- availability of appropriate professional support for counselling employees and where necessary, following formal referral, giving progress reports to the managers. Depending on the available occupational health staff training, resources and expertise this professional support may vary in its provision between the occupational health department and outside specialists or agencies
- a forum for monitoring, reviewing and improving the working of the alcohol policy.

Drug abuse

In many respects, the same principles concerning prevention and rehabilitation apply to drug abuse as to alcohol abuse. However drug abuse can sometimes pose greater difficulty in recognition and management especially because of the wide diversity of harmful agents and the range of occupational circumstances in which they may present. Moreover, the illegality of much drug taking adds a special dimension, at least from the point of view of managers.

Case history 9.10

A 26 year-old nurse was referred to the occupational physician because of doubts about her fitness for work. No specific details were identified in the referral letter although on enquiry the physician was told that she concentrated poorly, and seemed to forget instructions that she had been given and was slow in her work. On history taking and physical examination no cause for concern could be found and the physician reassured the nurse and her manager accordingly, but expressed a readiness to review her, on request if necessary at a later date. About 9 months later she was suspended from duty having been caught stealing benzodiazepines and other drugs from the ward. During disciplinary hearings it was claimed that she had become dependant on drugs after having been given anxiolytics when she was younger following the death of a parent. Extenuating circumstances were accepted and she did not lose her job. She was eventually rehabilitated in collaboration with a psychiatrist.

This was a near miss situation in so far as the worker's job and career were concerned, and in the circumstances she was fortunate not to be dismissed or even reported to the police for theft. If the environment had been such as to encourage the worker to have sought help on her own accord, or if the physician had suspected the diagnosis and asked the correct questions she might not have come within a hair's breadth of damaging her wellbeing for life through disgraceful dismissal from her job as a nurse. As with smoking and alcohol abuse, the abuse of drugs should be on the workplace agenda for health. Information and counselling should be to hand. However, there are some work circumstances where possession of certain substances or biological evidence of their consumption constitute automatic grounds for summary dismissal, for example in pilots. In these situations the monitoring and enforcement should not be associated with the function of the occupational health service, since this could hinder the effectiveness of that service in contributing to health promotion in the workplace.

Case history 9.11

An occupational physician was newly appointed to a firm that manufactured controlled drugs. The firm had a policy, stipulated in the contract of employment of each worker that possession of one of those drugs would result in instant dismissal without notice. In order to enforce this, workers could be searched without warning and some white collar employees were constituted into search teams for either gender. The physician discovered that the nurse had been assigned to a search team although never called to participate in one – indeed no search had been carried out within recent memory. The physician advised the factory manager that it was inappropriate for occupational health staff to participate in what was a purely disciplinary and enforcement role, while at the same time attempting to engage in health promoting activities, including availability for confidential counselling. The manager accepted this and the nurse was removed from the roll of search team members.

Similar considerations to the above would apply in the case of urine testing for drug abuse in conjunction with a disciplinary policy; this is not the responsibility of the occupational physician. However, where the occupational physician has control over the use of tests which determine the presence of toxic agents or their effects on the body (as in the measurement of gamma glutamyl transferase in a case of alcohol abuse), these tests may have a role if used in confidence with the worker's knowledge and informed consent.

Stress

Stress has been defined in a number of ways and the range of stress management techniques is even wider still. Essentially what most people understand by 'stress' is a physiological or psychological response to external stressors that goes beyond what is accepted as normal. Perhaps 'strain' would have been a better word and an analogy with a rubber band appropriate. Limited external stresses produce a response, a 'strain', which beyond a certain point becomes disproportionate and beyond the capability of the elastic properties of the subject. In the prevention of stress there are two poles of attitude. The prevailing one is usually to focus on individual behaviour by support and advice, to help coping with the stress. The second is to alter or reduce the outside stressors so as to reduce the stress. While not dismissing the former, the doctor in industry should concentrate, and focus employers' and employees' attention on the latter. This is however easier said than done, especially since stress is usually multifactorial.

Case history 9.12

A 53 year-old computing officer came to consult the occupational physician after her manager had informally suggested that some form of counselling or stress management advice might help her. The employee was tense, anxious and distressed because she had found progressive difficulty in keeping up with increased work demands. The unit was due to merge with another and she was uncertain of the consequences that this might have on her employment. She had some slight difficulties with vision because of severe myopia and a retinal detachment which had been treated, but this in itself was not a major problem, provided she could work at her own pace. Her manager who was involved in a later meeting said that she had become increasingly withdrawn into simple repetitive tasks while allowing a backlog of important requests to accumulate. The physician expressed the opinion that an adequate and sustained improvement in her well being would best be achieved by a change in her work plan and responsibilities. This was difficult to arrange but she was eventually given responsibility for the induction training in keyboard skills and basic computer training for new members of staff. This was a fairly circumscribed job with a steady and relatively predictable load and which was well within her skills and resulted in continuing useful employment and well being. A few years later her duties were changed again because of a reorganisation and she developed an anxiety neurosis. This together with some worsening of her vision prompted a premature retirement on ill-health grounds.

Case history 9.13

A senior manager telephoned the occupational physician and sought a consultation away from their usual workplace. He complained of headache, heartburn, anxiety and tiredness, and with difficulty in falling asleep. He said that he had increased irritability with his close colleagues and family, and that his libido had decreased. He had reached the conclusion that his symptoms were stress related. There had been many changes in the organisation, including the introduction of productivity targets expected of his unit and he had to transmit these stresses and expectations to his juniors. This placed him in internal conflict. Together with a number of his peers he was uncertain about the consequences of reorganisation in which it was rumoured that one or more of them would be made redundant from their current jobs. Physical examination was normal. Further discussion permitted him to identify various occupational stressors, unfortunately over which neither he nor the physician could exercise significant influence, especially since he did not wish any other people involved. The physician's reassurance that the symptoms were not an indication of some other underlying pathology provided some relief. The value of coping strategies such as allocating specific time and place for work and domestic activities was discussed and the physician provided him with further written information relating to other sources of advice.

The above cases illustrate some of the common occupational stressors which may affect even the most senior employees in an organisation. Sometimes individual employees are reluctant for their particular issues to be taken up by the physician in a way in which they might be identified and possibly be labelled as 'not coping'. However the physician can progressively build up a picture of the health of the organisation after seeing a number of workers with common problems. Retrospective review of the case records of the other employees from the same workplace might identify others with similar mental symptoms and sickness absence patterns may be worse than the norm. On the next workplace visit the physician could probe the organisational structure, bearing in mind the important determinants of stress illustrated in Fig. 9.2. Diplomacy and communication skills are then invaluable and essential tools. The physician should suggest to the senior manager that sickness absence and problems with performance generally might yet worsen. A responsible and open manager should be willing to explore the organisational determinants of stress and try hard to remedy them. Such an approach is more likely to result in lasting benefit to the workers and the organisation than the hiring of a stress consultant to lecture on individual coping strategies.

Different people vary in their responses to outside factors, be they psychological or otherwise, and therefore exhibit different degrees of vulnerability. As stated in Chapter 5, the role of the physician in relation to the workplace is to help ensure its safety, as far as is reasonably practicable. However many difficulties present themselves. Thus with agents such as noise and respirable dust, it is generally the case that the more there is, the worse it is for everybody, while on the other hand, psychological stressors may affect different people in opposite directions. For example tasks such as in information technology, which require a specific but limited degree of skill and knowledge, might be stressful to an employee who is set in ways and habits and is finding difficulty with coping. It could also become stressful to a keener, motivated employee who easily masters the skills, but for an opposite reason, in that the latter may become frustrated at not being able to progress and use his or her initiative and control over the programmes being dealt with. Although Fig. 9.2 has listed a range of occupational stressors, the reader should also consider causes of stress which are not included in it. Thus unemployment is a very important direct cause of stress, while indirectly the fear of losing one's job is a similarly serious stressor. Moreover physical ill health, family and other social problems, especially lack of support can add to occupational factors in provoking or exacerbating stress reactions.

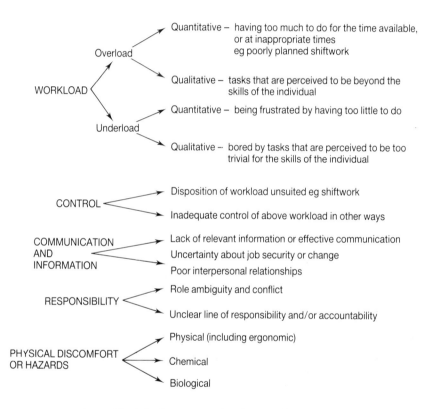

Fig. 9.2   Some occupational causes of stress

Immunisation

Immunisation as a means of promoting health can be an important tool, although of more relevance for some workplaces than others. It can fulfil the following purposes:

- it can protect the employee from ill health that may be a specific consequence of work, e.g. administering BCG (Bacille Calmette-Guerin) to

mortuary workers, or active hepatitis B immunisation of laboratory workers handling blood samples.

- in some situations, immunisation besides fulfilling the above function can also protect the health of members of the public besides employees eg immunisation of surgeons against hepatitis B
- immunisation may also offer protection unrelated to specific work risks e.g. immunisation against influenza virus

Immunisation policies like all other issues in health promotion should not be looked at in isolation but as part of an overall strategy and given correct priority

Case history 9.14

An occupational physician who was new to a particular workplace received a postal reminder inviting the repeat annual ordering of influenza vaccine. Further enquiry revealed that it was custom for all the workforce to be offered influenza vaccine once a year and approximately one third accepted. The physician's assessment of the workplace identified various respiratory hazards and indeed that some workers suffered from occupational rhinitis and/or asthma. The physician's advice to the manager and to the safety committee was that steps should be taken to control respiratory hazards in the workplace and that influenza vaccine should only continue to be offered (in line with the current Department of Health guidelines) to individuals at a particularly high risk such as those suffering from cardiac or pulmonary disease.

Case history 9.15

A nurse contracted hepatitis B. This coincided with national publicity on the risks of this disease for health care workers and the advantages of immunisation. Several individuals, work groups and managers made representations for immunisation and this was authorised at the highest level of line management. Some employees such as physiotherapists and radiographers were getting immunised while others, like nurses in gastrointestinal endoscopy suites were having to wait their turn. This was paralleled by inconsistent policy and advice on the disposal of sharp implements and on the management of exposures. After some effort a concerted policy was introduced. This gave summary advice on the risks of hepatitis B and allied infections, on the means of reducing these risks through appropriate workpractices, and on categorisation of employees into groups with different degrees of risk. Immunisation was then publicised and offered first to those in the highest risk group (including clinical departments of gastroenterology); after the first round was completed in these, it was then offered to groups at lesser occupational risk. Those groups deemed to be at a risk not significantly different from the general population e.g. health authority administration, and secretarial and clerical staff were not offered immunisation.

The above cases reinforce the need to put immunisation in its proper context, as part of an overall plan appropriately targeted and ranked in priority. Good information systems need to be in place to record which groups of employees have been targeted, have had appropriate information and education, have been offered immunisation, and the date of its administration. Arrangements for recall and review need to be similarly effective and efficient.

Diet, weight reduction and exercise

There is good epidemiological evidence that diet is an important determinant of health. Some characteristics of the Western diet appear to be associated with an increased risk of coronary heart disease and cancer of the large bowel and probably other diseases. However there is still some scientific debate on issues such as recommending an increase in the proportion of polyunsaturated fats in the diet. In general, however it would be appropriate for the occupational physician to offer the following advice.

- Reduce the total fat and oil in the diet with particular reduction of animal fats (in meat or in dairy products) with a relative preference to vegetable oils and fish oils
- Encourage high fibre plant foods such as beans, other vegetables and fruit
- Maintain an adequate intake of protein of vegetable and animal origin (but relying on fish, lean meat and low fat dairy products)
- Reduce overall intake of high energy foods, especially reducing intake of refined carbohydrates and alcohol.

Obesity is associated with an increased risk of some diseases, notably coronary heart disease, although there is probably not a direct causal link between the two. Moreover in individuals suffering from back pain and other musculo-skeletal complaints or other conditions affecting exercise tolerance such as certain heart and lung diseases, reduction of weight to the normal range can bring about a welcome improvement in symptoms.

Appropriate exercise undoubtedly improves well being and increases the cardiovascular, respiratory and muscular limits of tolerance to further activity. The extent to which exercise, completely independent of other factors, may reduce morbidity or mortality from say, coronary heart disease is unclear. Generally speaking graded isotonic (kinetic) exertion is a preferable activity since it does not impose a sudden strain on the musculo-skeletal or cardiovascular system. The redesign of jobs and work practices discussed in chapters 5 and 8 so as to reduce cumulative or acute musculo-skeletal injury can complement exercise programmes by providing work which is safer, involves less load but more appropriate movement in manual handling. While some workplaces do provide exercise facilities on site, and these are to be welcomed, they should come low down on the list of priorities after all reasonably practicable means have been employed to make the workplace safe.

In promoting health through altering lifestyle factors such as exercise, diet and hence body weight there is always the prospect of ending up by 'preaching to the converted'. However, as with stop smoking campaigns, workers in peer groups can help each other attain common goals. Nevertheless, as exemplified by case history 9.5, any campaign approach should be paralleled by an opportunisitic individual approach, in tandem with other health improving measures, notably health protection at work as illustrated in Fig. 9.3.

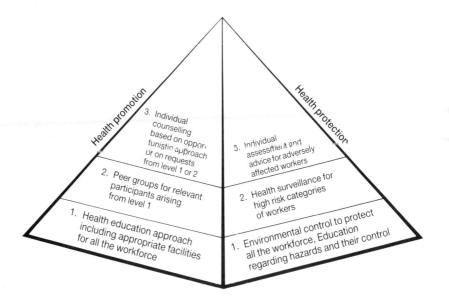

Fig. 9.3   Different levels and aspects of health promotion and heath protection in the workplace

Screening for non-occupational disease

This is an important subject that poses various questions:

- what for?
- why?
- at what cost?
- who?

Additional, complementary issues of scientific validity have been considered in Chapter 3, pages 70 and 73. Unfortunately 'screening' can become a bandwagon with a momentum of its own regardless of whether the essential criteria for scientific validity have been fulfilled. This is particularly true for diseases which are emotive or common, like cancer (e.g. breast, cervix) and coronary heart disease.

Case history 9.16

A 50 year-old security officer presented himself to the occupational health department asking whether a 'cholesterol test' might be on offer. He did not have any cardiac or vascular symptoms although he complained of 'heartburn' which was relieved by antacid tablets. His father had died at the age of 64 from pneumonia against a background of chronic lung disease while his 75 year-old mother was alive and well with no history of cardiac disease. He smoked 15 cigarettes a day since his early twenties and drank an average 10 pints of beer per week. He was normotensive and not overweight, and the rest of his physical examination was normal. The relevance of various lifestyle risk factors in general and particularly with regard to his lifestyle was explained by the occupational physician. He accepted that his smoking history presented a higher risk than that which might be related to blood cholesterol level. Cholesterol measurement was not pursued but he resolved to attempt to stop smoking and, to ensure his alcohol drinking remained under control and to engage in regular exercise. He succeeded in reducing his smoking considerably, although not stopping altogether.

Employees who seek advice about screening tests believe that these are proven markers for health risks and that, implicitly, knowledge of these may help reduce their risks. The health professional should listen to the employee and seek to understand the motivation behind the request, and then proceed to assess all the health risks and place them in the right order of priority. This should be followed by advice about reducing risks which are well recognised and which are important for the individual, before dealing with those which are speculative. Thus for instance, in case 9.16, the issue raised was that of cholesterol screening. Authoritative reviewers, after a critical appraisal of the evidence, have concluded that for the general population blood cholesterol screening and lowering does not reduce mortality and is unlikely to prevent coronary heart disease while being associated with other morbidity. Anxiety resulting from the screening, and adverse effects of treatment which may follow, are often inadequately catered for when balancing the risks and benefits of screening.

Case history 9.17

A 32 year-old executive was found to have positive dipstick screening test for haemoglobin in his urine in the course of a 'routine' medical examination in industry. A repeat test was also positive and he was referred back to his general practitioner with a letter indicating the results of this. A further urine test carried out by the GP was followed by a referral to a urologist, intravenous nephropyelography and cystoscopy. He was told very little about the purpose and the results of these tests. Besides the physical discomfort, he and his wife were very anxious about the proceedings and the implications. Eventually he was told that no abnormality had been found and remained physically well, although with the anxiety that he might have had something which had been missed.

So-called 'executive medicals' are widely practised in some sectors of industry. Good evidence that they constitute a cost effective way of promoting health at work is lacking and one wonders whether they are more of a status symbol whereby the recipient can demonstrate to colleagues how highly he or she is prized by the organisation. Various reports, mainly from North American companies, have suggested that initiatives to improve lifestyle coupled with health screening appear to reduce the medical bills for which the firms are responsible. However, there are hardly any well designed and executed scientific studies that have measured the effectiveness of health promotion in the workplace either in terms of improved health or productivity.

10

Ethics, communication and audit

Summary

The professional and ethical responsibilities of the doctor in industry to the individual worker, especially as regards confidentiality, consent and the duty of care are essentially no less than those applicable to other physicians. However, the doctor's duties to all employees within the workforce also entail a responsibility to give essential advice on fitness, safety and related health risks to the employer, and care must be taken to observe appropriate ethical principles in so doing. Particular attention should be paid to communication between the workplace doctor, professional colleagues and managers and employees. Thus the independent and politically neutral stance of the occupational health service is understood by all and its role in providing a healthy and safe workplace facilitated. Doctors in industry should aim to improve the quality of medical advice and the effectiveness and efficiency of the service through appropriate forms of audit in conjunction with clinical colleagues and co-workers.

Introduction

This chapter deals with three important facets of all medical practice which are often inadequately dealt with in medical textbooks. Although they are best learnt through experience under supervision, the reader is offered guidance about the general principles underlying the occupational physician's code of professional conduct, especially in relation to the workplace, quality of work and about advice and interaction with workers and others. Moreover, the practice of occupational medicine presents problems and dilemmas specific to this specialty which warrant particular attention and are therefore highlighted here.

Ethics

The fundamental doctor-patient relationship as enshrined in the Hippocratic oath applies in occupational medicine just as it does in other branches of medicine. The Faculty of Occupational Medicine's booklet on ethics for occupational physicians is essential reading. The main tenet, namely that the physician's prime concern is the health of the patient, who here is defined as the employee for whom the doctor has responsibility, is paramount. In occupational medicine this must include the obligation to do all within the physician's power to ensure the prevention of ill health in all the workers for whom he has responsibility, whether they consult him as individuals or not. The physician must of course also be concerned with the patient's social well-being. Generally speaking, prevention of ill health or restoration of health achieves this end too but this is not necessarily always the case.

Confidentiality and Consent

The physician is normally bound to keep in confidence all that is disclosed in the course of his relationship with the patient. However, there may be rare exceptional circumstances, in occupational medicine as in other specialties, where this obligation is not absolute but after careful thought may have to be limited. The terms of consent that apply to a consultation between an employee and an occupational physician should be explicit. When an employee is referred by the employer to the occupational physician, the latter should confirm these terms along with the purpose and plan of the consultation. Thus, it should be pointed out that the employer will be advised impartially on matters of fitness to attend work, to perform it satisfactorily and safely, and on the risks to health from work. All other matters remain in confidence between the physician and the employee.

Case History 10.1

A worker whose job entailed driving goods within and between various sites of a firm was referred to the occupational physician on account of repeated multiple short absences usually attributed to abdominal pain, dyspepsia, diarrhoea and vomiting. The worker's breath smelt of alcohol and after close questioning by the physician, it transpired that he had a serious alcohol problem and not infrequently drove at work while still under the influence of drink. He did not wish the physician to disclose this fact or the implications of it to his manager. The physician explained that his responsibility to the worker and his colleagues required him to advise the manager "that the worker is temporarily unfit to drive for medical reasons. This unfitness is not necessarily permanent but would be reviewed after 4 weeks. He remains fit to carry out other portering duties." The cause of this unfitness was not disclosed to the manager. A programme of alcohol counselling was commenced and after a further two reviews the physician advised the manager that the worker could resume vocational driving.

This example illustrates a common ethical problem in industry where an individual's abuse of alcohol can endanger himself and others. Many companies recognise this problem by having a written policy agreed by management and unions to deal with alcohol and drug abuse, providing appropriate opportunities for rehabilitation (see Chapter 8).

Case history 10.2

A foundry worker engaged in a non-ferrous foundry was being seen by an appointed doctor for the purposes of health surveillance in relation to his exposure to lead. His tasks in fettling included the use of hand held vibrating tools so as to remove excess metal from the castings. The occupational physician incidentally elicited symptoms of vibration white finger. He sought the employee's consent to advise the employer so that the employer could take appropriate remedial steps as well as reporting the occupational disease to the Health and Safety Executive. The worker asked whether the physician could guarantee his continuing employment without adverse changes in his status and earnings. Obviously the physician could not do this and the worker denied his consent for his employer to be informed.

Many workers fear, sometimes justifiably, that they will be discriminated against if they develop an industrial disease. They may therefore be very reluctant to allow a doctor to inform the employer of their condition. This may in turn lead to delays in preventive measures being implemented. Bearing in mind what you have read in Chapters 3 and 4 about the investigation and management of occupational diseases, what steps would you now have taken?

The physician suggested that he could speak to a medical colleague in the Health and Safety Executive's Employment Medical Advisory Service (EMAS) to present the problem in confidence and seek help discreetly. The worker agreed to this, and agreed to the occupational physician communicating his concerns to the general practitioner. After an appropriate interval, an official of the Health and Safety Executive made a 'routine' visit to the foundry, assessed exposure to vibration and made appropriate recommendations to the employers.

If the physician had advised the employer of the diagnosis, then the employer would have been legally obliged to report this to the Health and Safety Executive (under the Reporting of Injuries, Diseases and Dangerous Occurrences Regulations – RIDDOR). As with industrial accidents so also with disease there is evidence of under-reporting. If the physician has reason to suspect that this may be happening, then he should discuss his suspicions with medical colleagues in the Employment Medical Advisory Service of the Health and Safety Executive.

Occupational Health Records

The occupational physician is the custodian of clinical records and access to these is limited to clinical staff (physicians and nurses). Clerical staff in the occupational health service must have the confidential nature of these records stressed and give a commitment to respecting this confidentiality when they join the service before being allowed the access that is necessary for them to perform their duties. It may bear repeating to managers and to workers that even though the employers may own the case notes, in the same way that they may own everything else in the firm, the notes are in the secure custody of the physician and nurse and their contents will not be disclosed to the employer without the individual worker's informed consent. Similar considerations apply to clinical data that are stored electronically. Statutory obligations must be complied with, specifically those under the 1984 Data Protection Act such as the need for registration and the entitlement of individuals to access to data held on computer about them. Security measures, limitation of access and explicit documents to confirm this are particularly important where systems are shared or accessible through means of electronic communication, or where linkage is required, say with environmental data monitored by an occupational hygienist.

The doctor in industry should generally be prepared to discuss the contents of the occupational health records with the worker they concern. However, for this and other reasons, it may be useful to have the record subdivided. Thus, for example, separate sections should be devoted to pre-employment assessments, consultations following self- or management-referral and statutory health surveillance. Even in the last mentioned, a distinction may need to be made between the purely clinical data such as symptoms questionnaire or lung function tests on the one hand and a record of exposure, physician's conclusion and other basic information that constitutes the statutory 'health record' – as defined for example by the Control of Substances Hazardous to Health regulations (see Chapter 5). Under the Access to Health Records Act, patients will have access to various categories of health records, notably those within the National Health Service. Even though this might not apply to records in private industry, it is always good practice for the doctor in industry to keep records which he would not be ashamed of if 'discovered' by due legal process.

Legal disclosure of occupational health records can pose serious dilemmas – with or without consent. An important distinction must be drawn between a request for clinical records from a solicitor and a court order for disclosure of specified documents. The latter must be complied with or the physician may incur unlimited penalty if found to be in contempt of court. In the case of a request from a solicitor, the accompanying written consent of the worker concerned is essential. However, even with the worker's consent, there could be complications. Thus, some parts of the occupational health record of the individual may bear no relation to the occupational injury or illness in respect of which litigation is in progress. Rarely the names of other employees involved in a particular incident or exposure may appear in the record of the index worker and might need to be masked in any copy made. One situation in which there does not yet appear to be a clear consensus arises when a worker's solicitor asks for release of the worker's clinical record with the worker's consent while this consent is denied to the employer's solicitor. Understandably, the employer and his legal advisers may feel unfairly frustrated in that they are denied the information they need to respond to the worker's solicitor in anticipation of a possible Industrial Tribunal hearing or a Civil Action in a Law Court. One possible solution is to point out that the employer technically owns the clinical record. While this does not confer the right of access to the clinical record, it can entitle him to deny it to others. A consent by the worker for the relevant parts of the clinical record to be made available to solicitors on both sides could then resolve the impasse.

There is one specific exception to the rule that the occupational physician must disclose a report to the court in response to a court order or to the worker's solicitor with his consent. This arises when the occupational physician is specifically asked to see the worker and advise solely for legal purposes. Usually this request arises from the firm's solicitor. The physician must explain the special nature of this request to the worker and that neither the worker nor the worker's solicitor will be entitled to see the report but that it will be a privileged communication to the firm's solicitor.

Ethical relations with the general practitioner and other physicians

The role of the doctor in industry does not ordinarily extend to treatment of disease, prevention of ill-health that is not work-related nor the provision of a 'second opinion'. Thus the treatment which an occupational physician undertakes should be limited to emergency measures whether specific to occupational medicine (as described in Chapter 4) or otherwise. In any case the general practitioner should be informed of this as soon as practical and reasonable. Although limited administration of non-prescription therapeutic agents such as minor analgesic agents, emollient creams etc. need not warrant special attempts at liaison with the general practitioner, any other treatment of consequence should be agreed. Referral to a specialist in another discipline should ordinarily only be undertaken with the agreement of the general practitioner, except in an emergency. The role of the occupational physician in the prevention of ill-health and the promotion of health in those respects which are not strictly work related is discussed in Chapter 9. Advice of proven merit such as exhorting the worker to stop smoking is not likely to be contentious between medical practitioners and indeed should be encouraged. However, the implementation of other steps such as cervical screening should await an opportunity for the general practitioner to voice his opinion, or veto, especially as such matters may form part of the general practitioner's contract of employment. The occupational physician has a duty to advise a worker as to the possible health effects of his work or the implications of his health on his fitness for work. Of course, he need not refrain from giving such advice before consulting the general practitioner although the occupational physician should be cautious and circumspect in his statements if it is apparent that there is a divergence of opinion between him and the general practitioner. This is particularly germane when dealing with the small minority of patients who attempt to manipulate differences between their medical advisers. Finally, it should be stressed that the ethical constraints in relation to consent apply just as much to ethical relations with the general practitioner as with anyone else. Thus a worker might not wish his general practitioner to be aware of aspects of his medical history which could prejudice his chances of getting life insurance cover. Occasionally workers may have misgivings about the security and confidentiality of information disclosed to the general practitioner. The occupational physician may discuss these concerns with the worker and even try to allay them or find a reasonable compromise. Eventually though, the worker's wishes must be respected, however irrational they may appear. Similar considerations apply to ethical relations with other physicians.

Case history 10.3

> A 47 year-old hospital laundry worker was referred to the occupational physician under the hospital's alcohol policy. She had a deteriorating performance and attendance record and had been noted to be smelling of alcohol at work. When assessed by the occupational physician, she gave a history of heavy alcohol consumption and a past history of jaundice. Further assessment revealed Hepatitis B antigenaemia and macrocytosis, as well as biochemical abnormalities consistent with alcoholic liver disease. She refused permission for the occupational physician to advise the general practitioner on the grounds that the practice receptionist was a neighbour of hers.

This provides a real dilemma for the occupational physician. The patient is clearly ill and in need of help because of her alcohol abuse. Action is necessary which can hardly be concealed from the general practitioner indefinitely. Fortunately the employer had an alcohol policy which would allow a management programme to be instituted and which would protect the patient's job in the hope and anticipation of a successful outcome. But what should the occupational physician do about telling the general practitioner?

> After discussion with the patient about her anxieties, the occupational physician suggested that the general practitioner could be spoken to in strict confidence over the telephone. The patient agreed that the occupational physician could do this and moreover agreed to take part in an alcohol rehabilitation programme.

Risks to health from work

This subject is dealt with in detail in Chapters 2–6. The doctor in industry must be objective and impartial when assessing the risks to health from work. He has a responsibility to inform, assist in interpretation and advise management, the individual workers concerned, and their legitimate representatives about these risks. He must openly fulfil this duty of care to all concerned and remember, and remind others, that it is a greater duty than any contractual obligation to secrecy.

Ethical dilemmas

There are bound to be situations where guidelines do not provide explicit answers to an ethical dilemma. Yet there are very few circumstances in occupational medicine where a doctor has to advise or act without the possibility of time to think. Therefore, an occupational physician who might be in some doubt as to the 'correct' action should seek the advice of a senior colleague known to them personally or within an appropriate academic or professional organisation (such as the Faculty or the Society of Occupational Medicine).

Communication

Language of communication

The doctor in industry needs to develop special skills in communication. Skills at assessing workplace health risks, clinical acumen with patients and advice on management of problems are only of limited value if the doctor cannot 'get the message across". The role of the physician may include communicating an assessment of, say, a health effect as a consequence of work to a semi-literate unskilled worker, to a medical colleague (usually the general practitioner) and to a professional manager. Although the underlying principle to be communicated may be the same, the detail of the content and the language used may vary – although the physician should never be pompous or patronising in any case. It is essential for the physician to be familiar with the language used by the employees and employers in describing their tasks, their raw materials and their products. There is no substitute for frequent workplace visits to achieve this, although reading of relevant literature such as chemistry textbooks or process handbooks may help.

Although in the first instance many communications are verbal, there are many circumstances where the written word is essential. Thus, for example, formal referrals from a manager to assess a worker should include an explicit written statement of the problem as perceived by the manager, the evidence for it, and the advice required from the physician. This has been discussed in more detail in Chapter 7. This is particularly important where matters of great potential consequence to the worker are concerned such as consideration of ill-health retiral, or assessment and advice in connection with alleged alcohol or other substance abuse.

Another circumstance when written explicit advice is certainly warranted arises when a physician has evidence of a significant health risk as a consequence of work. The observations leading to this conclusion and specific remedial advice should be stated. If management procrastinates or prevaricates unduly in the face of a substantial risk, words to the effect that, in the physician's judgment, the risk warrants alerting the enforcement agency concerned (usually the Health and Safety executive) and the firm's insurers can result in a flurry of activity where all else has failed. These trump cards should, however, be used judiciously since perseverance and persuasion are usually preferable tools.

Main channels and content of communication

The doctor in industry should make it clear from the time of his appointment that all employees as individuals have direct access to him or her (often through the medium of the occupational health nurse) and that they are available for confidential consultations. Communication with appropriate managers is important. Thus a physician who has access to the factory manager is more likely to influence a change for the better in working conditions for the employees than one who is relegated to communicating with a junior member of the personnel department. Where the quality of line management is good and effective, it is probably better to liaise with the appropriate manager, rather than the personnel officer, about working conditions in his department or the problems of an individual worker. In some workplaces referrals from management are channelled through the personnel department. This can be useful if the quality of line management is inadequate and inconsistent criteria are used for referral to the physician. However, if this is the case, the physician should invest time in explaining the role of the occupational health service to the managers and in insisting that workers are clearly and fully consulted when referral is contemplated.

It follows from what has been stated earlier that since the prime ethical responsibility of the occupational physician is to the worker/patient, the communication between the two is of the utmost importance. At the end of the consultation, the employee must be informed of the doctor's conclusions even when the worker has been formally referred by the employer for advice from the doctor. A minority of occupational health services have a policy of providing the worker automatically with copies of their advice to the employer while any letters of referral from the employer are correspondingly copied to the worker. In any case the physician should always confirm with the worker the reason for the referral and explain what questions are being posed and what advice will be given in response. Many or all of the following elements should feature in the information provided by the occupational physician to the employee after making a clinical assessment:

- the nature of the clinical problem (if there is one) and the occupational implications – in so far as attendance, safety, performance and fitness
- important causative or contributory factors
- the likely severity and duration of the above
- what steps should be taken by the worker and the employer as appropriate to reduce the adverse consequences
- how certain the physician is of this advice
- what the physician will be saying, why and to whom
- any other reasonable advice or information which the worker wishes either spontaneously or in response to an invitation from the physician.

Communication with the general practitioner

In the vast majority of cases in which an employee asks or is referred to consult with the occupational physician, there is no need for the general practitioner to be consulted in advance. Some guidelines may be offered to exceptions to this. Thus, for example, if a worker has been off sick for a prolonged period and the general practitioner's sickness certificates suggest a serious organic or mental illness which may affect the worker's physical or emotional fitness to come and be seen, then the two doctors should probably liaise first. Once the occupational physician has seen a worker in consultation, there are circumstances when advice to, or other communication with, the general practitioner is usually warranted with the worker's consent. These include situations where the occupational physician's assessment and plan:

- has important implications for the worker's employment – such as a recommendation for ill-health retirement
- requires cooperation with the general practitioner – say for the purposes of organising a guided rehabilitation to work, or referral to another specialist or agency
- require further information which the worker might not be able to relate reliably such as the result of relevant investigations, drug history, severity of past psychiatric illness
- could result in education or information for the general practitioner relevant to the management of that worker/patient or to other workers such as by identifying risks to health from work or circumstances in which recurrent problems may be expected.

Communication with the Safety Committee and others

An important forum for the doctor in industry to communicate with both employers and employees is the Safety Committee. In the United Kingdom the provision of a Safety Committee is an explicit consequence of the Health and Safety, etc. at Work Act (1974) and the relevant guidelines also state that the occupational physician should be an *ex officio* member. Unfortunately, many Safety Committees are anodyne and effete bodies in which employers are represented by a junior member of management and employees by shop stewards, or union apprentices aspiring to this and with little training in health and safety matters. Nevertheless, the active contribution as outlined below by an enthusiastic doctor can improve considerably the value of the Safety Committee, and its contribution to the health and safety of employees, as well as enhancing his standing in the organisation. The physician's role on the Safety Committee should be that of an independent expert witness, not a representative of either party nor a chairman, adjudicator or arbitrator. It is up to the employer's and employees' representatives to reach agreement on how to control the risks to health from work. The physician's contribution should include formal reporting to the committee on relevant health problems within the workplace, summary accounts of the results of health surveillance of groups of workers, and responding to requests for specific advice from the committee. The doctor should advise the committee and assist it in its interpretation of current or proposed legislation (such as European Community proposals for directives). Important or controversial articles in the scientific or lay press that may be relevant to the firm in question should be explained to the committee. It may also be appropriate for the occupational physician to present a regular, say yearly or 6 monthly, report of activities, plans and targets to the committee, highlighting the major, strategic issues rather than being drawn on trivial items like the siting of washhand basins or fire extinguishers! In summary, active contribution to the Safety Committee without fear or favour is an essential part of the responsibilities of the doctor in industry. Physicians who do not undertake this and who allow themselves merely to be summoned to attend Safety Committee meetings only at management's behest so as 'to reassure the workers' end up being treated by the workforce at best with misgivings and at worst with suspicion and contempt.

Finally, a physician who works for a large firm or one with the potential for special and serious risks to the health of its employees should make the effort of establishing links with the Health and Safety Executive, relevant services and specialists at the local hospital and local general practitioners.

Audit

Audit has been defined as 'the systematic critical analysis of the quality of medical care. This may include, for example, the procedures used for diagnosis and treatment, the use of resources and the resulting outcome and quality of life for the patient.' Audit is relevant to all medical specialties and is gaining importance worldwide as part of the need to provide quality of service to the consumer and additionally prompted in the UK by recent changes in the National Health Service. There are various reasons why audit is particularly relevant to the practice of occupational medicine. First doctors in industry practise in isolation (as distinct from say hospital 'firms' or group general practices) and therefore formal attempts at getting together for the purposes of audit are important to ensure quality of care. Second, such doctors may not be fully accredited specialists and some of them, especially part-timers, are not engaged in any formal training programme. Audit can serve a very useful educational role, particularly for these physicians, by guiding them in better ways of managing common problems. Until recently, only about one half of practising UK occupational physicians engaged in audit fulfilling at least part of the above quoted definition and about one in 5 undertook audit activities approximating the full scope of audit as relevant to occupational medicine. There is however both a need and a desire among many occupational physicians to undertake audit and this section is intended to offer some guidance, although not a fully comprehensive account of the subject.

Classification of Audit

Several definitions, types and taxonomies of audit have been described, some of which require clarification for the reader. Thus, for example, some authorities prefer to use the term 'clinical audit' rather than 'medical audit' to highlight the need to involve other health care disciplines, notably occupational health nurses. On the other hand the 'clinical' adjective may tend to restrict the audit to the quality of care for the individual client/worker within the narrow confines of his clinical (Greek: *kline* = couch or bed) consultation. At this level, audit of the quality of assessments, communication and advice and of the individual outcome is very important for the purposes of continuing education of the health care professional as well as to ensure that quality of care for the individual is paramount before other quantitative performance indicators are embarked upon. At a higher and wider organisational level, audit should cover the effectiveness and efficiency of the service. *Effectiveness* is defined as the extent to which a specific intervention, procedure, regimen or service, when deployed in the field, does what it is intended to do for a defined population. *Efficiency* measures the effects or end-results achieved in relation to the effort expended in terms of money, resources and time.

When classified along another dimension, audit can be subdivided into audit of structure, process and outcome. Structure deals with the quantity, type of resources available and organisational framework. Process deals with what is carried out by way of assessment, advice and other intervention in relation to the worker. Outcome measures the results of the intervention by the occupational physician or occupational health service, such as reduction in morbidity or in health risks.

Choosing topics for audit in occupational medicine

The product of the possible topics needing audit and the possible means of accomplishing this for each topic is legion. The following guidelines should help a reasonable initial choice to be made. The topic to be audited should be locally common, or of high health risk or high cost in other ways and timely in its relevance. A preliminary review of the reasons for referral to the occupational health service, problems identified at consultations, 'accident" rates, and sickness absence rates, all major resource commitments of the occupational health service, should reveal many possible topics for audit. Alternatively, a random review of consultation records as outlined below has the merit of being simple and of selecting common reasons for consultation. It is essential to have a standard against which to compare the observed practice. Many activities undertaken in occupational medicine do not have a wide enough consensus or a solid scientific basis to serve as a 'gold standard' and it may not be rewarding to audit these in detail especially if there is additional local divergence on, say, the means of rehabilitating workers with musculoskeletal injury or on the extent of counselling for psychological stress. Nevertheless basic information relating to health records, nationally agreed protocols on say vaccination, or proformas such as those in Appendix 5 can be useful starting points in comparing observed practice with a standard. Topics should be chosen in which there is likely to be the need and the means for improvement in practice following comparison with the standard, the implementation of change and where the audit itself is cheap and simple. Thus the audit should seek to be cost effective by improving outcome and efficiency by education and changes in practice, at least initially. Audit is an iterative process of cycles which should result in an improvement and eventually sustained assurance of quality in particular areas while identifying needs and methods of audit in new areas (Fig. 10.1).

Methods of audit

In certain situations especially of an educational nature (trainer and trainee) or in a hierarchical context (chief physician and his juniors), occupational physicians meet to discuss and approve the conduct of their work. However, this is not an adequate system for audit since it involves only certain professional relationships and the subjects or case records covered are literally at the choice of either party. One means of more formal audit, especially of the process of occupational medical care, starts with the random selection of a small number of consultation records sampled from a serially kept day book. These are then shared out between the participating physicians such that each acts in turn as auditor or has his consultation note audited. The auditor reviews, in private, the consultation record against a proforma with key issues highlighted, perhaps assisted by a set of explicit criteria where these have been agreed. Subsequently at an audit meeting, the auditor presents a

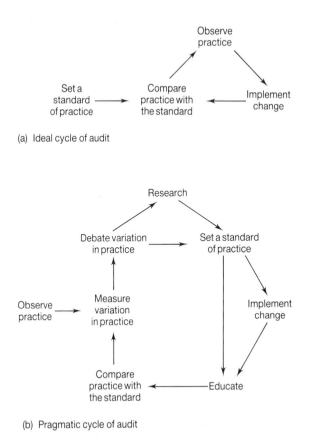

(a) Ideal cycle of audit

(b) Pragmatic cycle of audit

Fig. 10.1 The cycle of audit and related activities in occupational medicine

brief verbal account of his assessment of the consultation record and this is usually followed by a short debate. Neither the identity of the physicians nor the employee is minuted but a short summary of relevant points discussed and agreed actions is kept. These minutes are retained and can be used as confirmatory evidence of the audit and so as to assist the pursuit of remedial action. The detailed proformas can then be destroyed. The following tables illustrate some points in the proformas that may be useful as a guideline for the reader. Appendix 5.1 relates to a general proforma applicable to all occupational medical consultations. An important cause of referrals to occupational physicians is sickness absence and assessment of fitness to continue or to resume work and guidelines for a proforma to assess this are shown in Appendix 5.2. Various clinical problems can be encountered in occupational medical practice but two of the commoner ones relate to back pain and to mental health problems. Guidelines for proformas for the audit of these consultation records are shown in Appendices 5.3 and 5.4 respectively.

In some organisations such audit by peer review of process has been usefully widened to include other occupational health professionals, notably nurses, and this merits the wider description of 'clinical' rather than 'medical' audit.

The benefits of this form of internal peer review audit can be illustrated by the following examples resulting from actual meetings.

Case history 10.4

> A series of consultations had been carried out for the purposes of assessing continuing fitness for work of a porter. Eventually this culminated in a recommendation for ill-health retirement. It was noted that there was very sparse documentation of objective signs of physical impairment and this was debated by the various participating physicians.

What do you think are the minimum requirements for a decision on ill-health retiral? Do they include the likelihood of incapacity of attendance at work, of performing work satisfactorily, of doing it safely, or of all three factors? Does the incapacity have to be permanent? Would you rely solely or exclusively on the patient's history? To what extent can your assessment be objective and repeatable? (Chapter 7 may provide some of the answers.)

As a result of the audit of this case, an educational update on objective measures of physical impairment such as the assessment of lumbar spinal flexion, distraction and other clinical techniques was organised for the clinical occupational health staff. The functional requirements for this particular job were also discussed and agreed with the employer.

Case history 10.5

> A 36 year-old nurse was referred to the occupational physician with a history of multiple episodes of sickness absence and unacceptable behaviour at work. A previous hospital admission had suggested that her symptoms may have been related to alcohol abuse. The occupational physician had deemed her fit to return to her duties and reviewed her once. The notes were sketchy and the results of the examination were not recorded. The peer group felt that more detailed assessment, record-keeping and further review was warranted when there was evidence of alcohol abuse. Guidelines for further management of such cases were agreed.

The increasing availability of computer facilities in occupational health services should assist considerably in the development of quantitative and on-going methods of audit of process and of outcome. The data required must be collected accurately and prospectively, easily retrieved for the purposes of the audit but otherwise securely kept. Thus strategic objectives and specific targets may usefully be set, for example, for the uptake of a vaccination programme, and for acceptable time intervals for sickness absence or other referrals for specific problems to the occupational health department, and acceptable time intervals for the assessment and response by the occupational physician.

Whatever topics are audited or methods used, it is important for the audit to be non-threatening, educational and interesting for all participants as well as being objective, repeatable, effective and efficient in its aims.

Appendix 1

The reporting of Injuries, Diseases and Dangerous Occurrences Regulations (RIDDOR) and diseases prescribed for Industrial Injuries Benefits under Social Security Regulations

Riddor

These regulations put on the *employer* the responsibility of reporting to the Health and Safety Executive certain accidents and diseases. The accidents and dangerous occurrences are described in Chapter 6. It should be noted, however, that a number of conditions that might be regarded as diseases are reportable under accidents if that is what caused them, for example toxic pneumonitis following inhalation of irritant gas or a slipped disc while lifting a heavy weight, would not be reportable under the list of diseases but should be reported under accidents if they result in over 3 days of absence from work.

The following are included in the list of reportable occupational diseases:

Disease		Numbers reported 1987–92
1.	Poisoning (acrylamide, arsenic, benzene, beryllium, cadmium, carbon disulphide, dioxan, ethylene oxide, lead, manganese, mercury, methyl bromide, nitrochlorobenzene, nitrogen oxides, phosphorus)	62
2.	Chrome ulcer	62
3 & 4.	Oil/tar folliculitis or acne	6
5.	Oil/tar skin cancer	10
6.	Radiation skin injury	15

Disease		Numbers reported 1987–92
7.	Occupational asthma	292
8.	Extrinsic allergic alveolitis	34
9.	Pneumoconiosis	22
10.	Byssinosis	5
11.	Mesothelioma	48
12.	Asbestos lung cancer	1
13.	Asbestosis	34
14.	Nickel lung cancer	-
15.	Leptospirosis	45
16.	Hepatitis (blood exposure)	136
17.	Tuberculosis (hospital or animal contact)	44
18.	Infection due to work with pathogens	87
19.	Anthrax	–
20.	Bone cancer (ionising radiation)	–
21.	Blood dyscrasia (ionising radiation)	3
22.	Cataract (electromagnetic radiation)	9
23.	Decompression sickness	174
24.	Barotrauma	1
25.	Nasal sinus cancer (wood, leather, nickel)	5
26.	Hepatic angiosarcoma (vinyl chloride)	–
27.	Urinary tract cancer (naphthylamines, benzidine, etc.)	15
28.	Vibration white finger	470

Several points can be made from this list. First, it excludes some of the most common diseases (dermatitis, deafness, upper limb strain disorders) and includes several very rare ones. Second, it is acknowledged that there is substantial under-reporting, and few employers (or doctors) will be aware of the need to report, say, oil folliculitis or barotrauma to the ear. Third, some conditions do seem to get reported, such as vibration white finger and the infectious diseases, these latter probably because the doctors who diagnose them have residual memory of earlier regulations related to public health.

The Health and Safety Commission, in its annual report in 1993 drew attention to under-reporting and gave preliminary estimates of the prevalence of occupational disease from the 1990 Labour Force Survey. These suggested that the common work-caused diseases are:

Work-caused disease	Approximate prevalence 1990
Back disorders	290000
Other musculoskeletal	260000
Stress/depression	110000
Deafness	105000
Lung disease	60000
Skin disease	60000
Upper limb strain	50000
Asthma	30000

These figures represent responses to a questionnaire, and are therefore estimates based on individuals' views of their own health. While therefore likely to represent an over-estimate of the size of the problem, they go some way to redress the balance.

Prescribed diseases

This list of diseases for which Industrial Injuries Benefit is claimable, assuming the patient has worked in an appropriate occupation, is kept under regular review by the Industrial Injuries Advisory Council, who from time to time recommend the addition of other conditions caused by specific occupations. The list includes the following:

Disease	New cases in 1991
Pneumoconiosis	447
Asbestosis	330
Byssinosis	7
Farmers' lung	5
Asthma	293
Mesothelioma	519
Asbestos lung cancer	55
Other lung cancer	6
Asbestos pleural thickening	149
Deafness	1041
Dermatitis	432
Tenosynovitis	556

Disease	New cases in 1991
Beat knee, elbow	187
Hepatitis, TB, leptopirosis	5
Poisonings (as for RIDDOR)	4
Cancers (bladder, nasal sinus, skin)	17

It should be noted that these figures represent successful claimants, that is those who not only have the disease, but also are considered to be disabled by it.

Appendix 2

Occupational exposure limits

The principal route of exposure to substances hazardous to health is inhalation of dust, fume, particles and fibres from the work environment. Using evidence from a variety of sources (historical, laboratory, epidemiological), occupational exposure limits have been agreed for a small percentage of substances used in industrial processes. These limits are either not to be exceeded and designated as maximum exposure limits, or are levels to which employees may be exposed without risk to their health and are recognised as an occupational exposure standard. As such they can be regarded as adequate control of that substance for the purposes of the COSHH Regulations as far as exposure from inhalation is concerned.

The reference period for occupational exposure is either long term (usually over an 8-hour period) as a time weighted average (TWA) or a 10-minute short-term exposure limit (STEL). These time-scales allow for variability in the effects of exposure to substances hazardous to health depending on the nature of the substance and the degree of exposure. Some substances cause harmful effects which are only manifest after repeated or prolonged exposure. These will be controlled by reference to the TWA, e.g. benzene, wood dust. Other substances produce harmful effects after only brief exposures, either single or repeated, and therefore require, in addition to the TWA, a short-term limit which applies to any 10-minute period throughout the working shift. Examples are formaldehyde, trichloroethylene.

Occupational Exposure Standards

In 1992, 473 substances were assigned an occupational exposure standard (OES). For a substance to be assigned an OES it must meet the following three criteria:

1. The available scientific evidence can identify a specific concentration, averaged over a reference period, at which substances are unlikely to be harmful to health if employees are exposed by inhalation day after day.
2. Exposures to concentrations higher than that specified in 1 (above), and which could reasonably occur in practice, are unlikely to produce serious short or long term effects on health over the limited time in which they would occur.

3. Compliance with the OES as defined in 1 (above) is reasonably practicable. The only consideration in setting the level is the protection of the health of the employee.

Maximum Exposure Limits

In 1992, 36 substances were assigned a maximum exposure limit (MEL) meaning that the available evidence on the substance does not satisfy either the first or second criteria for an OES and exposure to the substance has, or is liable to have, serious health implications for workers. Alternatively, although the substance meets the first and second criteria for an OES, socioeconomic factors require a numerically higher value if the control measures required are to be regarded as reasonably practicable to implement.

Serious health implications include both the risk of serious health effects to a small population of workers and the risk of relatively minor health effects to a large population. MELs are most often allocated to carcinogens and to other substances for which no threshold of effect can be identified. A MEL is therefore the maximum concentration of an airborne substance, averaged over a reference period, to which employees may be exposed by inhalation under any circumstances and is specified, together with the appropriate reference period, in Schedule 1 of the COSHH Regulations.

These exposure limits, together with limits for hazardous substances which have their own regulations, e.g. asbestos and lead, and appendices relating to man-made mineral fibre, cotton dust, asphyxiants, rubber fume and dust, grain dust and potential carcinogens, are published by the Health and Safety Executive in *EH40, Occupational Exposure Limits,* which is updated annually. This document also contains useful lists of other Health and Safety Executive publications and guidance notes on the methods for the determination of hazardous substances (MDHS) series: the environmental hygiene (EH) and medical series (MS): and a list of documents pertinent to the COSHH Regulations.

Tables 1 and 2 in EH40 list the occupational exposure limits relating to adequacy of control of exposure by inhalation as required by the COSHH Regulations. However there is additional annotation identifying substances

- for which there may be significant exposure by absorption through the skin (SK)
- which are capable of causing respiratory sensitisation (SEN)
- which are new additions (NEW)

Examples of substances with a maximum exposure limit, occupational exposure standard, or annotations are listed in the following table.

Examples of Occupational Exposure Limits

Substance	Formula	Long-term exposure limit (8hr TWA reference period)		Short-term exposure limit (10minute reference period)		Notes
		ppm	mg/m³	ppm	mg/m³	
Maximum Exposure Limits						
Benzene	C_6H_6	5	16	–	–	
Formaldehyde	HCHO	2	2.5	2	2.5	Sen
Isocyanates		–	0.02	–	0.07	New
Nickel	Ni	–	0.5	–	–	New
Silica	SiO_2	–	0.04			New
Styrene	$C_6H_5CH=CH_2$	100	420	250	1050	
111 Trichloroethane	CH_3CCl_3	350	1900	450	2450	
Trichloroethylene	$CCl_2=CHCl$	100	535	150	802	Sk
Vinyl chloride	$CH_2=CHCl$	7	–			
Wood dust (hard)			5			Sen
Occupational Exposure Standards						
Acetic acid	CH_3COOH	10	25	15	37	
Acetone	CH_3COCH_3	750	1780	1500	3560	New
Ammonia	NH_3	25	17	35	24	
Carbon black	C		3.5		7	
Carbon dioxide	CO_2	5000	9000	15000	27000	
Glutaraldehyde	$OCH(CH_2)_3CHO$			0.2	0.7	
nHexane	C_6H_{14}	20	70			New
Malathion	$C_{10}H_{19}O_6PS_2$		10			Sk
Ozone	O_3	0.1	0.2	0.3	0.6	
Toluene	$C_6H_5CH_3$	50	188	150	560	Sk
Welding fume			5			
White spirit		100	575	125	720	
Xylene, all isomers	$C_6H_4(CH_3)_2$	100	435	150	650	Sk
Zinc oxide, fume	ZnO		5		10	

Appendix 3

Sources of information

This appendix lists sources of information which provide helpful information and guidance to the occupational physician who is seeking to solve a particular problem in clinical practice. Occupational health information is scattered throughout the literature in several subject areas. It is found in general as well as specialist medical journals and in a range of biomedical science journals.

Textbooks

General and Encyclopaedic

Hunter's Diseases of Occupation, 8th edn., P.A.B. Raffle et al. (eds); Edward Arnold, London 1994.

Handbook of Occupational Medicine. Robert J. McCunney (ed.); Little, Brown and Company, Boston/Toronto 1988.

Occupational Health Practice, 3rd edn. H.A. Waldron (ed.); Butterworths, London 1989.

Lecture Notes on Occupational Medicine. H.A. Waldron; Blackwell Scientific Publications, Oxford 1990.
A good account of occupational disease.

Fitness for work: the medical aspects. F.C. Edwards, R.I. McCallum and P.J.Taylor (eds); Oxford University Press, Oxford 1988.
Essential reading for all occupational physicians.

ILO Encyclopaedia of Occupational Safety, Volumes 1 and 2.
International Labour Office, Geneva 1983.
This two-volume encyclopaedia remains a useful reference source. The articles are written by an international panel of experts and therefore may not necessarily reflect current practice in the United Kingdom.

Occupational Medicine. Carl Zenz (ed.); Year Book Medical Publishers Inc., Chicago 1988.
This is the major large American textbook which covers the whole range of occupational medicine, the wider aspects of occupational health and practical management issues.

Environmental and Occupational Medicine. William N. Rom (ed.); Little, Brown and Company, Boston 1992.
The best current textbook of occupational disease.

Specialist Topics

Occupational Lung Diseases, 3rd edn. W.K.C. Morgan and A. Seaton; Saunders, Philadelphia 1994.

Essentials of Industrial Dermatology. W.A.D. Griffiths and D.S. Wilkinson (eds); Blackwell Scientific Publications, Oxford 1985.

These books cover in some detail two areas which commonly give rise to clinical problems in occupational medicine.

Occupational Hygiene

Monitoring for Health Hazards at Work. I. Ashton and F.S. Gill; Blackwell Scientific Publications, Oxford 1992.
This is a useful practical manual on monitoring hazards in the workplace. It is an essential book for anyone who occasionally has to undertake simple monitoring surveys in the absence of an occupational hygienist.

Toxicology

Casarett and Doull's Toxicology. The basic science of poisons, 4th edn. Mary O Amdur, John Doull and Curtis D Klaassen (eds); McGraw Hill, Hightstown NJ 1991.

Patty's Industrial Hygiene and Toxicology, Volume 1 (General Principles) Volume 2, (Toxicology), Volume 3 (Theory and Rationale of Industrial Hygiene Practice), 4th edn. George D. Clayton and Florence E. Clayton (eds); John Wylie and Sons, New York 1991.
This is a reference book, currently being updated, which provides detailed information on all aspects of worker and workplace health and safety. Whilst it is written for the American market, the principles are universally applicable.

Epidemiology

A basic knowledge of epidemiology is important when dealing with the health of groups of people as well as to allow critical appraisal of published papers. The books selected provide the necessary introduction to the subject.

Searching for Causes of Work-Related Diseases. Jorn Olsen, Francis Merletti, David Snashall and Karl Vuylsteek; Oxford Medical Publications, Oxford University Press, Oxford 1991.

Epidemiology in Medicine. Charles H. Hennekins and Julie E. Buring: Little, Brown and Company, Toronto 1987.

Updating services

There are now a number of useful cumulative loose-leaf publications which enable the reader to keep up to date with new and current issues. They include:

> *Croner's Substances Hazardous to Health*
> *Croner's Health and Safety at Work*
> *Kluwer's Handbook of Occupational Hygiene*

from Croner Publications Ltd, Kingston, Surrey.

Primary journals

The following is a list of peer-reviewed journals which publish articles on occupational medicine. Articles will occasionally appear in other journals and so the list, which is derived from *Index Medicus* and is in alphabetical order, should not be considered exhaustive.

> *American Industrial Hygiene Journal*
> *Annals of Occupational Hygiene*
> *Archives of Environmental Health*
> *Occupational and Environmental Medicine* (formerly *British Journal of Industrial Medicine*)
> *International Archives of Occupational and Environmental Health*
> *Journal of Occupational Medicine*
> *Journal of Toxicology*
> *Occupational Medicine*
> *Scandinavian Journal of Work, Environment and Health*

The *British Medical Journal* and *The Lancet* publish leaders, review articles, original papers and case reports which are of relevance to occupational medicine.

The following two non-peer reviewed magazines are useful in keeping the reader up to date with changes and proposed changes in legislation as well as medical and technical issues.

Occupational Health, published monthly, is a magazine intended for Occupational Health Nurses.

Occupational Health Review seeks to bridge the gap between management and medical and scientific issues. Included are notices of changes in the law, review articles, news and meeting reports.

Abstracting services

An abstracting journal lists, in a convenient way, the contents of a number of other journals and provides a brief summary or abstract of the papers indexed. This information enables the user to assess the potential value of the reference. *Index Medicus* and *Excerpta Medica* are likely to be the chosen publications.

Index Medicus covers about 2700 medical journals. Each monthly issue consists of articles indexed by both subject and author.

Excerpta Medica covers 3500 medical and scientific journals but excludes nursing, dentistry and veterinary science. However, it includes a number of books, conference papers and dissertations. Each issue contains a number of abstracts arranged in broad subject groups followed by an index of authors and subjects.

Selected Abstracts on Occupational Diseases is published quarterly from the Department of Health and Social Security Library. It is compiled by the research librarian to the Industrial Injuries Advisory Council. Abstracts are listed under the headings of the effects of physical agents, biological agents and chemical agents, cancers and respiratory diseases. There is also a detailed subject index.

On-line databases

The widespread availability of desk top computers, modems and communication software has made the on-line searching of databases more widely available. This service is available in many university, medical school, and teaching hospital libraries where skilled help may be available from the librarians. The relevant databases for the occupational physician are:

> *Medline*
> *Excerpta Medica*
> *OSH-ROM*

Medline is the computerised version of *Index Medicus* and includes approaching a million citations from over 3000 journals. Searching is interactive with the user identifying needs by responding to a series of queries raised by a computer. Search may be by author, title, word, publication date, language, journal or a combination of these elements.

OSH-ROM is produced by Silver Platter. It contains three bibliographic databases that cover international occupational health and safety information. *HSE-line* is produced by the Health and Safety Executive. Most articles are cited by author, title, source, publisher and date. A large proportion of the citations include documents such as consultant reports and conference proceedings. It is particularly useful as it includes material not found in traditional journal sources. It also emphasises material relevant to United Kingdom practice. The other databases are *NIOSHTIC*, which is produced by the National Institute for Occupational Safety and Health (USA) and *CISDOC* which is produced from the International Occupational Safety and Health Information Centre of the United Nations International Labour Organisation.

Other databases are available for specialist subjects and information regarding these should be available from the librarians.

General information

The Health and Safety Executive (HSE) have established a public enquiry point for information about official publications, guidance notes, and changes in exposure standards. It is open from 9 am to 5 pm, Monday to Friday. The address is:

HSE Information Centre, Broad Lane, Sheffield S3 7HQ
Tel: 0742 892345; Tx: 54556 HSERLSG; Fax: 0742 892333

In addition there is a new service, HSE Free Leaflet Line, for callers wishing to acquire free leaflets which are also available from the above address.

HSE has 21 area offices located throughout the country in major towns. HSE inspectors are useful sources of advice as are their medical colleagues in the Employment Medical Advisory Service.

The National Health Service has approximately 70 consultants in occupational medicine throughout the country. They may be prepared to provide general advice regarding health problems and hazardous work situations. The Faculty of Occupational Medicine has a network of regional speciality advisors whose locations correspond to the National Health Service Regions. The Faculty of Occupational Medicine (Tel: 071 487 3414) and the Society of Occupational Medicine (Tel: 071 468 2641) may be able to help in identifying a local source of advice.

Appendix 4

Training in occupational medicine

New medical graduates are often completely ignorant of occupational medicine, yet most soon realise that some knowledge of the subject is desirable if their patients' needs are to be adequately served. Some will eventually wish to take on sessional work, usually from general practice, advising companies on health in the workplace. Others may wish to specialise in the subject.

For the nonspecialist, the best training option is a short course, and these are available throughout the UK. In 1994, the Faculty of Occupational Medicine is instituting an examination for a Diploma in Occupational Medicine, to be taken after attending some 20 days of instruction. Information on courses may be obtained from the Faculty at the Royal College of Physicians, 11 St Andrew's Place, Regent's Park, London or from local postgraduate deans. They range from full-time, through modular and day-release to distant learning.

For the intending specialist, there are career and training opportunities in the National Health Service, larger industries, the Health and Safety Executive and the armed services. There are also a very few academic posts. Training requires the completion of the normal 2 years general professional training, during which it is usual to obtain membership of a Royal College, followed by 4 years of specialist training. This must be in a post approved by the Joint Committee on Higher Medical Training and must have a supervisor who is appropriately qualified. Such posts are advertised usually in the British Medical Journal and through the Society of Occupational Medicine, 6 St Andrew's Place, Regent's Park, London. During the first two years of this higher training it is usual to attend a course of instruction and take the examination for Associateship of the Faculty of Occupational Medicine and, towards the end of the 4 years, to complete a dissertation for Membership of the Faculty.

Further details of training and examination syllabuses can be obtained from the Faculty at the address above.

Appendix 5: Audit in occupational medicine

5.1 Audit applicable to all consultations

Consultation Record Details

Was this consultation one in a series with his patient?

Employee Information

- Age
- Occupation
- Workplace
- Number of hours worked per week

Referral Details

Mode: e.g.
- Management
- Self
- Occupational Health Nurse

Reason: e.g.
- Pre-employment assessment
- Routine health surveillance
- Ill health retirement
- Other re fitness for work/sickness absence

Adequacy and legibility of information provided
Time interval between referral request and appointment

Recorded Assessment

- Legibility –   Identifiable signature/designation, Date
- Employee assessment
- History   –   Occupational
             –   Symptomatic
- Examination

Recorded Conclusion

- Specific diagnosis
- Occupational implications for the employee
- Follow-up plan for the employee
- Plan for workplace assessment

Recorded Communication

- Employee
- General Practitioner
- Employer

Summary of Clinical Problem

Other Information and Comments

e.g. - Alternative methods of management
      - Ethical and legal aspects
      - Any evidence of outcome

Points that merit to be minuted/action

5.2   Audit of consultations for sickness absence/fitness to continue work

Is employee on sick leave at the time of the index consultation?
If 'Yes' then how long for?

Recorded Referral Details

Does the referral:
- Specify a long term absence?
- Quantify the long term absence?
- Specify short term intermittent absences?
- Quantify the short term intermittent absences?
- Specify another problem concerning performance or safety?
- Include a relevant account of the employee's job/tasks, place and hours of work

Recorded Questions Posed and Relevant Responses

- Current level of fitness for work
- Likely date of return to work
- Specific limitations in redeployment of the employee
- Existence of any underlying medical conditions which may contribute to unsatisfactory attendance, performance or safety
- Likelihood of the employee to render regular and efficient service in the future
- Likely duration of any residual disability
- Advice on whether work could be affecting the employee's health
- Advice on rehabilitation

Outcome following Occupational Physician's Advice

5.3 Audit of consultations for back pain

History

- Onset – Timing
  – Symptomatic description
  – Precipitant
  – Precipitant as work related incident
- Reference to physiotherapy
- Assessment of activities relevant to occupation
- Aggravating factors/movements and limits of tolerance of activity
  – Occupational
  – Non-occupational
- Relevant past history (first/recurrent/chronic)

Examination

- Distribution of pain
- Local back signs
- Lumbar spinal flexion – General comment
  – Specific measure
- Straight leg raising
- Neurological features

Other Investigations

- Lumbar spine x-ray

Diagnosis and Conclusions

- Anatomical/Pathological/Aetological
- Statement of objective functional impairment
- Disproportionate behaviour/psychological overlay

Advice/Action

- Rest
- Activity
- Advice on fitness for work

- Physiotherapy
- Workplace assessment
- Occupational   –   Graded rehabilitation
                  –   Long term accommodation

Comments and Other Information

5.4   Audit of consultations for mental health conditions

History

- Onset   –   Timing
                  –   Symptomatic description
- Reference to drug therapy
- Occupation   –   Title and tasks
                  –   Qualitative workload
                  –   Quantitative workload
                  –   Timing of symptoms in relation to work
- Relevant past history
- Enquiry about mental symptoms
- Enquiry about somatic symptoms
- Enquiry related to possible substance misuse
- Enquiry about social support

Examination

- Mental state examination   –   Affect
                             –   Behaviour
                             –   Intellect/Other higher functions
- Other examination

Diagnosis and Conclusions

- Nature of condition
- Possible causative factors   –   Occupational
                               –   Non-occupational
- Other adverse health risks

Advice/Action

- Workplace assessment
- Advice on fitness for work
- Reduction of occupational stressors
- Reduction of other stressors
- Further professional advice/support

Comments and Other Information

Index